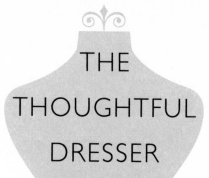

THE
THOUGHTFUL
DRESSER

THE ART OF ADORNMENT,
THE PLEASURES OF SHOPPING,
AND WHY CLOTHES MATTER

LINDA GRANT

SCRIBNER

NEW YORK   LONDON   TORONTO   SYDNEY

SCRIBNER

A Division of Simon & Schuster, Inc.

1230 Avenue of the Americas

New York, NY 10020

First Scribner edition April 2010

SCRIBNER and design are registered trademarks of The Gale Group, Inc.,
used under license by Simon & Schuster, Inc., the publisher of this work.

For information about special discounts for bulk purchases,
please contact Simon & Schuster Special Sales at 1-866-506-1949
or business@simonandschuster.com.

The Simon & Schuster Speakers Bureau can bring authors to your live event.
For more information or to book an event, contact the Simon & Schuster Speakers
Bureau at 1-866-248-3049 or visit our website at www.simonspeakers.com.

Designed by Mspace/Maura Fadden Rosenthal

Manufactured in the United States of America

1   3   5   7   9   10   8   6   4   2

Library of Congress Control Number: 2009043435

ISBN 978-1-4391-5882-1
ISBN 978-1-4391-5881-4 (pbk)
ISBN 978-1-4391-7164-6 (ebook)

For three generations of Ur women: Ziona, Ruth, and Lia.
Never knowingly underdressed

CONTENTS

THE
THOUGHTFUL
DRESSER

Dress has never been at all a straightforward business: so much subterranean interest and complex feeling attaches to it. As a topic, it is popular because it is dangerous—it has a flowery head but deep roots in the passions. On the subject of dress almost no one, for one or another reason, feels truly indifferent: if their own clothes do not concern them, somebody else's do.

ᐁᕝ ELIZABETH BOWEN

IN WHICH A WOMAN BUYS A PAIR OF SHOES

TWELVE YEARS AGO I saw a red high-heeled shoe from an earlier era. Glorious, scarlet, insouciant, it blazed away amid the rubber soles and strong cotton shoelaces as if to say, "Take me dancing!"

At night, when I cannot get to sleep, I sometimes distract myself by inventing its imaginary owner. I see her waking one morning in a foreign city, and as she raises the blinds on a spring day, the sun striking the copper rooftops, she realizes that she must go out *this very moment* and buy a pair of red shoes. A wide-awake girl in a white nightgown parting the shutters on a Paris day, drinking a cup of coffee, lighting a cigarette, thoughtfully smoking it before she quickly eats a roll, puts on her lipstick, and leaves the house.

Or I wonder, instead, if she is somewhat older—say, thirty-eight—in a gray wool coat and lines descending each side of her mouth, a small ruddy birthmark on the side of her right cheek, which she fruitlessly tries to cover up by curling her hair in waves below her ears, but the wind always catches it and exposes the strawberry stain. She is walking down a Prague street, a shopping basket over her arm, to the market to buy carrots, leeks, mackerel, and passes by chance a shoe shop, and there are the red shoes in the window—all by themselves on a little plinth raised above the lesser footwear, the price tag coyly peeking out from the base—and she has such a powerful urge to go in and try them on that that is what she does. Even though her husband, who is a little mean, would go mad if he saw how much they cost. He married her because of his jealousy and her birthmark: he could not stand another man to look at his wife.

The shoes fit. She empties the contents of her purse, counting out the coins and notes, and flees home with them tied up in a brown paper parcel, and hides them for several days at the back of the wardrobe. Not once does she think about her birthmark.

Or is she the Imelda Marcos of Central Europe, a rich, bored woman with countless pairs of shoes, a widow with a younger lover whom she will never allow to see her without a full face of powder, rouge, and lipstick? Or I think of a humble shopgirl or secretary who saved her wages for weeks circling past the shop, always fearing that by the time she had the money to pay for the shoes they would be gone.

I have tried to imagine the transaction in the shop in dozens of ways, and then the figure of a woman walking home (or driving, or taking a bus, a tram, a taxi), but whatever her station in life, her age, her figure, and her marital situation, the one thing I can be sure of is what she felt: that pleasurable frisson of excitement and delight when a woman makes a new purchase in the clothing department, and particularly an item as nonutilitarian as a pair of red high-heeled shoes.

Whatever her identity, I am certain she would have loved those shoes, or they would not have ended up where they did. She would have left them at home at the start of the journey if she couldn't stand in them.

The red high-heeled shoe exists. You can see it for yourself if you travel to Poland, drive a couple of hours west from Kraków, and visit the museum which is what remains of the main camp at Auschwitz (not Auschwitz-Birkenau, an extension, which is a couple of miles away, the site of the Final Solution against the Jews). Auschwitz I was the administrative center of the death camp. It is a popular excursion for tourists and Polish schoolchildren who are taken there by their teachers to learn about history. I don't know if they do or not.

Behind one of the glass-fronted display cases lies a great mountain of footwear, found by the liberating army in a part of the camp known as Kanada, in January 1945. The goods collected from the deportees, when they arrived by train, were placed there to be sorted through and distributed to the civilian population of Germany. The pile of shoes is designed to be symbolic, representing the footwear of twenty-five thousand individuals from one day's activity at the camp, at the height of the gassings.

So someone arrived at Auschwitz wearing, or carrying in her luggage, red high-heeled shoes, and this shoe is all that is left of her. When I visited Auschwitz, I was transfixed by the shoe, for it reminded me that the victims were once people so lighthearted that they went into a shop and bought red high-heeled footwear, the least sensible kind of shoe you can wear. They were human, fallibly human, and like us; they took pleasure and delight in the trivial joys of fashion. This anonymous, murdered woman, who died before I was born, would surely have bought her shoes in the same spirit that I bought mine.

Apart from underwear, more fragile and temporal, shoes are the most intimate garments we wear. They are imprinted with the shape of our bodies. Looking at the shoes in the artfully arranged pile at Auschwitz, I saw not a monument, but fashion. The fashion in the late thirties for red high-heeled shoes. So you have genocide, and you have fashion, and genocide could not be more awful and serious and fashion could not be more superficial. Yet the woman who bought the shoes was not only a statistic of the Final Solution. Once upon a time, she liked to shop for stylish footwear.

Whenever I have bought expensive, painful, unnecessary shoes, I have thought about her, the now anonymous woman who arrived at the camp wearing the shoe (and its partner) or carrying it in her luggage. She was not anonymous then. She had a name, a life. Freedom, in its way, was the right to buy expensive luxuries, to own nice things. Fashion exists, whatever you think about it. It's everywhere, even in the gruesome relics of an extermination camp.

You can't have depths without surfaces. It's impossible. And sometimes surfaces are all we have to go by. In the case of the shoe in the camp, that's it, there's nothing else—not whether she was a good mother or a dutiful daughter or a medical student or a keen reader or a skilled chess player. The shoe is all there is, and it has its own eloquent language and says a great deal.

When, several months ago, I started to write about the red shoe in the pile at Auschwitz, I had a doubt about its authenticity. It was known by architectural historians that the displays at what is now the museum had been the product of tinkering by postwar Polish communist ideology, designed to illustrate the great antifascist struggle. The camp you enter as a visitor in 2009 is not the same camp that was liberated by the Soviet troops in January 1945. A lot of things have been moved about (to create a cafeteria, toilets, and gift shop), and it was always possible that the red shoe had been bought at a shop in Kraków sometime in the sixties and added by the museum's curators to create an effect.

A friend suggested that I ask the expert, Robert Jan van Pelt, who had written the definitive study of Auschwitz and its satellite camps, a book I had read several years earlier, before my own visit to Poland. Extremely nervous, I e-mailed him in Toronto, tentatively explaining that I wanted to check whether the red shoe was what it was purported to be and not a postwar fake. Expecting a dusty answer. How dare I reduce and trivialize the greatest crime of the twentieth century to a thesis on stylish footwear!

But almost at once I received a reply. Yes, he said, the shoe was indeed kosher, so to speak. But his wife, Miriam Greenbaum, had an additional question. Was I that Linda Grant who wrote sometimes about fashion, and if I was, would I like to meet a woman who had survived Auschwitz to become the great doyenne of Canadian style, the retailer who had introduced to a conservative female market such designers as Versace, Armani, Ferre, and Missoni? Indeed had survived because of her own vanity, out of a young girl's desire to, as she says, "look pretty"? And because she knew how to take one piece of clothing and turn it into another?

I traveled to Toronto to meet Catherine Hill, a woman who understood fashion and who understood darkness. For many days I sat with her in her apartment while she, with great courage, revisited places in the past so painful to be forced to remember, but always shared with me her stupendous insight into fashion and the great designers she knows, throwing a great searchlight on the questions I had been thinking about all those years. What fashion is, its significance, and why clothes matter—what happens when even clothes have been taken away from you.

For as Catherine Hill revealed to me, it is in the pleasure that we take in clothes that we are at our most elementally human. In clothes the story of the human race begins.

☙

In my own life, thank God, there has been no such suffering, only the usual disappointments and sadnesses we can all expect. Nothing truly terrible has ever happened to me.

When I look back I can detect the various periods through what I wore. I see myself at fourteen, wearing hideous clothes because I am both fashionable enough and conformist enough to *have to have* what everyone else is wearing whether it suits me or not. At nineteen, I'm a hippie, in maxidresses and a curtain of long hair, parted in the middle. At twenty-two, I exclusively wear clothes which are now called vintage but were then just secondhand or even "old"—1930s crepe de chine evening gowns, puff-sleeved blouses from the war. I bought them at Kensington Antique Market in London and scorned the browns, oranges, and huge collars of the era. At twenty-seven, a feminist, I'm in dungarees. In my early thirties, I have, briefly, a real job and a suit. In my forties, I gain weight and wear far too much black. In my fifties, I have rediscovered color and am starting to buy designer labels. This potted history is a time line of how I appeared to others and how I felt about myself. For as I had been brought up to believe, clothes matter. They matter for many reasons: because as you look, so will you be judged. Anyone arriving at a job interview wearing torn jeans and flip-flops should have learned that lesson when they received their letter of rejection.

But clothes are also about pleasure, as Catherine Hill so deeply understood from the word *go*.

⚭

One day last summer, at the moment of waking, I knew that I had to go out at once and buy new shoes. Shoes which fulfilled a function apart from walking. I wanted high-heeled shoes. Ridiculous, sexy, "I don't care how much they cost, I have to have them" shoes.

It is my habit always to trust the thoughts that flood my mind as I rise up out of sleep. The closer you are to the dream state, the more likely you are to receive the correct messages. The unconscious knows what it's doing and what it's talking about. If it tells you to go out and buy high-heeled shoes you can't walk in, there has to be a reason. I never pay any attention to those deceptive lightning flashes of brilliance from the lurid world of tossing-and-turning insomnia. They are worry thoughts, unlikely to enrich your existence.

As it happened, I had a hairdresser's appointment that morning. When it was over, I walked quickly down the street, full of the excitement and apprehension of the shopper who knows she is going to make a significant purchase. I was anxious because shoe shopping is no great pleasure for me, not compared with dresses and bags. I have inherited from my Eastern European immigrant ancestors wide feet, thick ankles, and heavy calves, legs developed in the womb to later hold up childbearing hips and bread-kneading arms. They are not my best feature, and no amount of exercise will ever fix the problem. A woman is born with good legs; if you don't have them, you can't get them however long you spend doing Pilates. There is no cure for dimpled knees. Growing up, finally, is about understanding that we are limited by our fate. There are unfulfillable dreams.

So shoe buying is always for me work, an ordeal. I go into the shop and see a pair of shoes I like and ask for them in my size, and of course they do not have them, or if they do, they don't quite fit, or the heels are so high I can't stand up without wobbling.

After working my way down all the shoe shops of the street with no luck, at last I came to a department store, which, like all large shops, feels to me when I enter as if I am pulling a building-sized fur coat around my shoulders, embracing and encompassing. A willowy Lithuanian salesgirl approached me and, appraising my terrible legs, silently handed me a shoe. She gazed in sorrow at my horrible ankles. Some time later, I descended the escalator carrying the shoe and its other half: high-heeled, black patent, peek-toe shoes by Dolce & Gabbana, with an oversized faux buckle. They lay swaddled in individual black cotton bags wrapped in black tissue paper, nestled in a lacquered black box.

For a whole day they sat like a pair of queens on a chair in my living room—burnished reflective leather monarchs. I couldn't take my eyes off them. Did I even deserve to wear them? They were the most expensive shoes I had ever bought, but I was prepared to measure them by a different scale of value: the amount of pleasure which I anticipated they would bring me, knowing that they were the *right* shoes.

Several days followed in which I waited for their first outing, when they would reveal their many secrets, such as whether they actually fit (or had I deluded myself in the shop, as I had done with a pair of Marni shoes the previous year, which cruelly cut into the instep after five minutes) and how long I could stand in them, given the height of those four-inch heels.

I would learn that the absolute maximum amount of time I can stand in my D&G shoes is about two hours, after which I have to sit down. I can only walk two or three blocks in them, but that is hardly the point, is it? I did not buy them to go walking, I have other shoes that fulfill that particular function. The D&G shoes possess a spectacular pointlessness. Aesthetically, they rise, *soar*, above their mundane purpose of protecting the soles of the feet from dirt and stones. They give me the self-confidence to look tall people in the eye. The black patent gleams and winks. The high heel makes a sexy arc. My back is straighter, my clothes hang better. But above all I'm making a statement, and that statement is, "Look at me."

Because when you are my age, born in the 1950s, there is nothing that people would like better than to pretend you are invisible.

And perhaps this is what my subconscious was trying to tell me when I woke that morning and knew that I *had to have* a pair of high-heeled, difficult, indeed impossible shoes. That the message was: *Be seen.* Be a presence in the world. For there is nothing worse than being a beige person, leading a beige sort of life. I mean, nothing worse for me. Others do not mind blending into the background; they crave anonymity. It suits them down to the ground. I have another point of view.

My unconscious did not warn me that it was reckless to spend so much money on a pair of shoes with the coming recession. It did not advise me to pay off my debts. It did not lecture me about making do, and mending. Although I don't follow the financial pages of the newspapers, and mentally switch off when I hear the words *Dow Jones* or *FTSE,* my unconscious pays close attention. It must be listening to the news on the sly because it knew that if there were dark times to come, at least I would have one pair of beautiful shoes to cheer myself up. For if you are poor, it's always best to give the appearance of the opposite, to inspire confidence—in one's self and others.

If we were heading into the Great Depression, I wanted to arrive there well dressed.

༄

For a long time I have been trying to get to the bottom of this relationship we have with our clothes and why we love or hate them and what they mean to us and how we are linked to them in all their intimacy with our own bodies. I have been thinking these thoughts not as a fashion historian or as someone capable of making pronouncements about style, or who can explain how Alexander McQueen cuts a jacket or how to put together a look. I once went to the Paris collections and gazed in incomprehension at the Dior show, the models lifting their feet like hooves, galloping along the runway at top speed like racehorses, and had to wait until the next day to buy the *International Herald Tribune* and have it all explained to me by fashion journalist Suzy Menkes. The *pleasure* of the Dior show—my own name in beautiful copperplate inscribed on a card actually glued to my numbered seat, the massed photographers with their lenses glittering under the lights, the intense beauty of the clothes—all suffused me with profound wonder, like a man who has been looking at the stars in his background through a pair of binoculars and is suddenly allowed to gaze at the universe through the Hubble telescope. But I didn't actually understand anything. I am not a fashion writer, just an amateur enthusiast.

I think about clothes and fashion in two ways. With the attention of the average person who simply wants to know what to wear next (no! not high-waisted pegged trousers!) and also with the interest of a writer who is curious about all our human dimensions, our comedy and our tragedy, our modest weaknesses and our occasional unexpected heroisms.

Writing and thinking about clothes is generally relegated to the fashion pages of newspapers and magazines or to the scholarly works of the costume historians. You only have to say the words *fashion pages* and you can see the mouth form a contemptuous expression. Fashion is lightweight, trivial, and obsession with appearance the sign of a second-rate mind.

So you might think that clothes are optional—marginal and irrelevant to the lives of most of us, something we can easily live without, as I can pass through my entire existence untroubled by the desire to go rock climbing, watching films starring the late Bruce Lee, making my own jam, or playing whiz-bang kill-the-baddies games on a console. Or reading a book by Terry Pratchett.

I consider it to be absolutely normal to care deeply about what we wear, and detest the puritan moralists who affect to despise fashion and those who love it. Who shrilly proclaim that only vain, foolish Barbie dolls, their brains addled by consumerism, would wear anything but sensible clothes made to last. As if appearances don't matter when, most of the time, they are all we have to go on. Or sometimes all that is left in the ruins of a life.

So I no longer take seriously those derisory accusations leveled against those who are interested in clothes. You might as well level them at Proust, Virginia Woolf, George Eliot—all of whom wrote about clothes and thought about clothes. I certainly won't take it from those men who judge and condemn women for the various failures of our appearance while simultaneously barking that only feeble shallow creatures such as women would pay any attention to how they look.

That is the great misogynist trick.

There are no known societies who do not adorn the human body, whether with clothing, jewelry, or tattoos. It's a given about the human race. You can even read the Bible, particularly the Old Testament, as an exercise in decoding the styles prevalent among Bronze Age men and women, the use of gold ornamentation, and the frequent futile demands by the prophets of women to spend less time thinking about what they wore. The great experiments of Puritan dress, in seventeenth-century England and its export to the new American colony, and China's utilitarian Mao suit collapsed within years of their introduction. Doomed to failure. People like variety in their clothes. They want the latest fashions. This is to do with the twin desires for pleasure and for change.

Clothes have been a constant in our lives since we lost our fur. We are born naked and stay naked for only a few moments until we are wrapped in our first clothes. In our small shoes, our little trousers and tops and shorts, until we grow out of them in leaps and bounds, and begin to develop our own ideas about what to wear—we have always got something or other on. Though we may be in rags, no one is ever totally naked. Mother Teresa said she could manage with a bucket and two saris. But not without *any* saris.

Looking out of the window, I don't see anyone who is undressed. There are only a few moments in the day when we are naked. We are naked in the shower and (but not even necessarily) when we have sex. The rest of the time we are always wearing something or other. I could spend all morning looking out of this very window, onto a main road and bus route, and examine what people have on, and speculate on why they have chosen those specific garments. Because they are on their way to work? Because they are delivering my mail? Because they are walking their children to school? Because they have a job interview or a hot date? Because they have absolutely no dress sense whatsoever?

Clothes matter; we care about what we wear, and not caring is usually a sign of depression, madness, or the resignation to our imminent death.

When the average woman looks in the mirror and sees herself more stylish, more beautiful, slimmer, her skin tone enhanced by the right colors, she can sometimes find it hard to live up to this person. The divide between the inside of your head with its private spaces and how you are seen by others can be intimidating. But not because you don't care. You care. We care about what we wear.

I don't believe people who tell me that they are not interested in clothes and do not care what they look like. I think they mean that they are not interested in fashion, and believe that following the trends is a waste of time. They look for comfort and a reasonable fit in the clothes they buy, and that will do. But such an attitude lies on the surface. There is something shallow about asserting it doesn't matter how you appear to others, because in your heart of hearts you know it isn't true. People want to look the best they can. They may not know how to find the clothes that fulfill this, they may regard the effort of doing so as too daunting, they might be frightened of the necessary expense, they might argue that they have no occasion to wear such garments or that the clothes don't go with their personalities. But it is simply untrue to say that if you take the average woman of average height and weight and income and wave a magic wand, fairy-godmother-style, and put her in a dress that makes her look beautiful, or a pair of jeans that fit perfectly, she will react with indifference.

When I watch the makeover shows (sometimes disagreeing profoundly with the outfits the guinea pigs have been given), I examine the expression on the faces of the women who have been transformed. I have seen shock and joy. I have seen women weep with happiness and freeze with fear or react angrily because they have been so altered beyond recognition that they no longer feel themselves to *be* themselves—a stranger looks back at them in the mirror. It is in the eyes of a woman who has been made over that you can observe at its most elemental the power of clothes and their capacity to unleash our emotions.

೦⁄೦

In the worst circumstances of your life, if you are left with nothing, the last nothing you own are your clothes. "I have nothing," said a survivor of the Chinese earthquake in the ruins of what was once a place, a town, a whole society. "I don't even have a rice bowl, just the clothes on my back." And the perennial boast of the successful immigrant is how they arrived in a country with nothing but the clothes on their back.

Society will allow you to starve to death and not lift a finger, you can die for want of medical attention, but you will not be allowed to go about naked. Public nudity is only one up from the incest taboo. You will even be dressed for the grave.

Clothes exist to keep us warm, to shield us from the wind, rain, and low-hanging branches. They protect us from various forms of social and religious shame: shame that we are exposing our sexual places, and embarrassment that we are revealing the existence of low-lying stomachs, man-boobs, flabby buttocks, and bingo wings—those waving appendages to the upper arms that attach themselves to middle-aged women.

Clothes are also adornment, they are pleasure, they signal our place in the world and send out highly important messages about ourselves. On the street, they are part of the aesthetic landscape. Trees, flowers, architecture, clothes.

The purpose of this book is to advance no thesis, to break no ground in the history or theory of fashion, but rather to explore what is already known but rarely thought about by the ordinary mass of humanity who is interested in fashion and might, quite wrongly, feel a little ashamed of this passion. Might fear that they are not going to be taken seriously. That in announcing this preoccupation they will have confessed that women are not really fully grown up; unlike our male counterparts, who have mature and adult preoccupations without which the human race could not survive, such as moving balls from one end of a grassy field to the other with the aid of the human foot.

꩜

There has never been a time in my life when I have not been interested in clothes. Even if I dressed badly or couldn't afford to buy what

I wanted. I would still look at other people and think, I wish I could wear that, but you should not look to me for a lesson in style and taste. I don't have the eye, that immaculate eye which knows how to put together an outfit, which understands that this color goes with that, or identifies a combination which makes a fabulous clash. I am more interested in how clothes and fashion make us feel.

Yesterday I went to see a man about a dress. The man was a designer, and the dress was to be worn at one of the most important occasions of my life, the black-tie dinner at which the announcement would be made of the winner of the 2008 Man Booker Prize. For which I was shortlisted. The only woman. I took a sea green dress and high heels to show him. The dress and shoes lay down and died under his derision, as if I had invited Saul Bellow to join a book club in which we were planning to discuss *Bridget Jones's Diary*. *Nothing* was right about the dress, including the haphazard stitching, he pointed out cruelly. He gave me another dress. This is what happens to movie stars at the Oscars.

I thought I knew what I liked and what suited me, but apparently I hadn't a clue, not when in the presence of one whose whole world this is. I am a total amateur, but that does not prevent me from taking an amateur's interest and recognizing that the people who bring us beautiful clothes are no less great artists than the people who bring us films and novels and paintings. They give us pleasure and transform us, even though we don't know how, and do not understand the concealed magic in the cut of a shoulder seam.

၉၀

How my own interest in clothes came about is deeply embedded in my family's history and my upbringing; it was as much a part of my world, growing up, as the flour that dusts the clothes of the miller's children.

I owe my superior private education entirely to the average woman's desire to have her hair shampooed, set, cut, permed, and tinted.

This was my father's business, and the money he made from it paid for me to attend a bluestocking school established in the nineteenth century to provide an academic education for the daughters of gentlemen. Though by the 1960s they let anyone in who had the cash and whose offspring could pass the entrance exam.

I was a great reader; I did almost nothing else but lie stomach down on my bed, precociously attacking books not meant for my age range, but because of my ambition to work my way through what I believed to be important (*Crime and Punishment* at age thirteen). I moved on to writing sensitive teenage poetry, while all the while haunting the little shops on Mathew Street in Liverpool which sold A-line minidresses. Shops the size of parlors, some still with coal fires. Now utterly vanished, and over their bones have been built the WAGs' Selfridges, Cricket.

Or turning the pages of the Biba catalog, desperate for an orange feather boa. Or unevenly applying Mary Quant eye shadow, Max Factor pancake foundation, masklike, and Rimmel mascara. Or studying photographs of Jean Shrimpton wearing Young Jaeger. Or considering how much less I would have to eat to have legs with a space between the thighs, like Twiggy.

Names clutter my recollection, shops and designers I never saw, only read about: Ossie Clark, Celia Birtwell, Alice Pollock, Jean Muir, Quorum, Mister Fish, John Stephen, Bus Stop, Hung on You, Granny Takes a Trip.

When I was a teenager, in the sixties, not to be interested in clothes was farcical, for to follow fashion was to know that you were alive in that decade of revolution and newness. Clothes were more than what you put on; they were the means by which you situated yourself in the present tense, and perhaps more important, at the time, the way you could be guaranteed to annoy or even horrify your parents. For we understood that we were the generation that had been born young and would stay young forever; growing old, as one's parents did, was a bizarre, mysterious lifestyle choice they had once fatally made—as if it had been their *intention* to have wrinkled skin and gray hair and spreading flesh, undiscussed illnesses and old-people's Crimplene skirts.

The first clothes I chose for myself, the first real outfit, was a brown turtleneck sweater, a denim skirt, and round-toed green patent shoes. I wore this ensemble to lunchtime sessions of the Cavern Club a few months after the Beatles had stopped performing there. I concealed the garments carefully in my school satchel when I left home in the morning. Then I would make my dental appointment excuses to the school secretary, get on the bus, go into town, get changed in a public lavatory, and stand in the queue with other truant twelve-year-olds to enter a warehouse which smelled of damp, decay, and extremely cheap scent.

I listened to bass guitars and echoey drums, the Hamburg Sound which came to us via the "race records" which black American merchant seamen sold in the pubs on the dock road and which were bought by the teenage John Lennon, who sat in his bedroom around the corner from my own, playing them over and over. The Mersey flowed hurriedly west, to join the Atlantic. You could smell and taste the salt air in the chords.

Then back to school in the middle of the afternoon to droop over *Ivanhoe*.

That was how it started. An expensive education paid for by the vanity of women, and a rebellious teenager who implicitly understood that clothes were the way she set herself up in opposition to her parents' wishes, the children of Eastern European immigrants. Content in the suburbs, they wanted nothing more than for their two girls to be dutiful daughters and wives. My mother was not an unfulfilled career woman. She liked shopping and gossiping with friends over coffee. Trailing around behind her through the shops, I received an apprenticeship in shopping and dressing. My mother knew what was in fashion and where you went to buy stylish clothes. On our annual visits to London there was always a visit to some little shop she had read about in a magazine where they sold handbags imported from Italy. She taught me that you had to keep your eyes and ears open, that you needed a strong visual sense and a good understanding of what did and did not suit you. I eagerly followed the instructions then rewrote them. In jeans whose hems I had deliberately frayed, barefoot, I looked like a beggar, a ragamuffin. *It's all the rage,* I raged. But my parents didn't understand a thing.

I would move on to even more incomprehensible choices: the Laura Ashley milkmaid look, which involved getting the train to Shrewsbury to buy sprigged cotton dressed with piecrust collars and matching pinafores designed to make you look as if you were churning butter in a late-nineteenth-century Welsh farmhouse. I wore that look for years on end until its feyness dropped out of style and was replaced by the hairy black Moroccan cloak I found in the Lanes in Brighton, the velvet embroidered Afghan dress with the little round mirrors that winked in the sunlight, and the round John Lennon glasses with the pink-tinted lenses.

Yet despite my parents' utter dismay at what I wore, despite my mother's fruitless pleas for me to just take a look at Young Jaeger, where they had fawn trews put together with a crocodile skinny belt and a coffee-colored turtleneck sweater (tending, already, you see, toward beige), they had wittingly instilled in me an innate understanding of the importance of how you looked and dressed. For as every immigrant knows, with the opportunity for complete reinvention, without a past, a history, in a strange land, how you look is what matters.

But all I had done was to evaluate what a girl of my age, in that period, should be wearing, and wore it. I wanted to be taken for what I was, an artistic bohemian who was as at home in the library as she was shopping in Carnaby Street.

When I try to look back at my life, when I try intensely to remember, and to understand who I once was, I find myself thinking about what I wore. Because these outer forms were a means of expressing something about what I wanted to be. I see years in which I dressed not to attract attention because I was so absorbed by writing that I wanted to be in a neutral zone. I see years when clothes ceased to be any kind of pleasure because of the fruitless struggle to find anything to wear. I see years in which I was a spendthrift, buying, buying, buying. I could write my autobiography in clothes from birth to present.

∽

But I am not just interested in myself. Thinking about clothes, what we wear and what other people wear, allows us to travel through time and space, to penetrate the thoughts and feelings of those long dead, or whose lives seem so baffling that we can scarcely believe them to be the same species as ourselves. When we look at dummies in a costume museum on which have been fitted outfits carefully preserved from the eighteenth century, we can admire the lace, the beads, the embroidery, but seldom feel that this is the kind of dress we might wish to wear ourselves, though designers are always taking inspiration from the past, Vivienne Westwood decking us out in mini-crinis.

Examining those bustles, whalebone corsets, hoopskirts, and ruffs, I don't see myself in a cloche hat, but I find myself thinking of the woman who once wore these garments, full of the passions I feel myself when it comes to trying on a new dress.

The people of other centuries seem so different to us that I think we would scream and go mad if we were suddenly dropped from a great height into, say, Silver Street in sixteenth-century London, where Shakespeare lodged for a few years with a family of "tire-makers"— makers of not wheel coverings but court headdresses. The stench of the streets, of the open sewers, would kill us. But through descriptive language we can make common cause with the past.

For people have written and thought about clothes ever since we could write and think. The Old Testament begins its story with how we first got dressed, blaming, inevitably, the need for it on the duplicity of women, and later laying down numerous rules and regulations on what God wants us to wear and how we are constantly aggravating him with our sartorial transgressions. Descriptions of the heathen peoples that the Jews must not resemble indicate that in biblical times there was a prevailing fashion for what would, several thousand years later, be revived as punk, with Mohawks, earrings, and tattoos.

In late October 2007, I started a little fashion blog. I had experienced the guilty pleasure, every morning, of logging on to my two favorite sites. Manolo the Shoeblogger, the extremely witty and intriguingly erudite website of an anonymous American whose tortured experiments with English syntax were a satire of both the Italian-born shoe designer Manolo Blahnik and the vacuous language of the fashion world. "Manolo loves the shoes!" he proclaimed. I took this Manolo, correctly, to be a persona (I would later enter an e-mail correspondence with its author in his nonfictional guise), but through his site, I started to awaken a hitherto dormant appreciation of what shoes can do for the personality, for the happiness of the moment, which led to the eventual purchase of my D&G black patent four-inch heels.

My other morning read was the Bag Snob, in fact two Chinese-American women of apparently lavish incomes, whom I initially believed to be fifty-something social X-rays, as Tom Wolfe puts it, Upper East Siders who sallied forth each morning to Bergdorf Goodman, followed by an extremely light lunch. It turned out one of them lived in a small town in Texas, the other in Boston, and they were old college friends now at home with young children, vicariously living through their handbag purchases, partly financed through their site's online advertising. Wow, they really knew their bags. Eventually, I would share and jointly consume two bottles of Veuve Clicquot with the Texan bag snob, in her suite at Claridge's on a visit to London. I held, for a few exciting moments, her latest Chanel bag.

On the Internet were thousands, probably millions, of women who were talking about clothes and about fashion. Some pored over photographs of celebrities, executing judgment on Paris Hilton's skirt and Victoria Beckham's shoes. Others scoured the shopping sites to put together whole outfits. Or they tried to give their readers the heads-up on the coming season's trends. Or, sweetly, they put up photos taken in their bedrooms of themselves modeling their latest purchase, and like a magic eye, you could see into the homes of complete strangers, and watch them experiment with the shaky beginnings of an identity in formation.

Eventually, I added a third site, that of the uncompromising Sartorialist, who simply took pictures of people on the street he considered to be particularly well dressed, and, usually without comment, allowed his readers to discuss what made their clothes work, or sometimes not.

And so, after some thought, I began my own blog. I began it as a way of thinking aloud, about this book, which I had already planned to write. I put on it quotations I had found about clothes and fashion, items from the news that interested me, my own frustrating quest for a dress with sleeves, which fell below the knee. In time I acquired a partner, a sidekick, "Harry Fenton," a friend with a sharp eye for middle-aged menswear and an almost perfect recall for the Mod styles of the mid- to late sixties.

Over time, the readers of the blog became a small but quite devoted community, whose comments and discussion were always intelligent, thoughtful, and extremely funny. I solicited their help as I was going along, writing and thinking about this book. When I asked American readers to share their own recollections of fashion after 9/11, they obliged with moving recollections of the days and weeks after those cataclysmic events, proving my thesis: that what we wear affects *every-thing*.

So this book's modest intent is to liberate its readers from the doubts and uncertainties that beset them when they start thinking about clothes or, worse, talking about them, and someone pipes up that they should concern themselves with matters more significant, such as the fate of the planet. Or the war in Iraq. Or the collapse of the banks.

We care about what we wear. If we don't we are fools. Only babies don't worry about what they look like, and only because no one has yet shown them a mirror.

Fashion must be the most intoxicating release from the banality of the world.

Diana Vreeland

THE ART OF
TAKING PLEASURE

LAST YEAR I went to an exhibition of the Golden Age of Couture at the Victoria and Albert Museum in London. The Golden Age was the decade spanning 1947 to 1957, between the launch of Christian Dior's New Look and his untimely death ten years later. Beyond Dior lay in waiting the boutique, and Bardot's observation that couture was for old ladies.

My mother was twenty-nine in 1947, a devotee of fashion, and though, with her petite figure, she was not really suited to the voluminous skirts of the New Look, she made me aware in my childhood of the elegance and glamour of those years. The furs, the jewels, the gloves, the hats. Observing her sitting at her kidney-shaped glass-topped dressing table, applying her makeup with a light hand, I learned that being a woman was something to do with clothes and cosmetics, and these activities were a sheer delight, to be taken seriously. By "seriously," I mean that you did them properly.

The V&A exhibition introduced me to some of the most fabulous garments ever made. Dresses, coats, suits by Dior, Balenciaga, Balmain, Givenchy, and Hartnell. Examining in one of the display cases a heavily beaded and embroidered ball gown, almost capable of standing up all by itself and heading off to the dance floor for a waltz, a friend exclaimed, "But who could possibly *wear* such a dress?" Peering at the details on the card next to it, I read aloud, "The Queen."

Yes, our dumpy, gray-haired monarch in the perennially oddly colored coats with matching bags and gloves, wore this once.

For those who are hazy about the history of fashion, on February 16, 1947, at his salon at the Avenue Montaigne in Paris, Christian Dior, already forty-two, a timid, plump, shy man, showed his first collection. His father owned a factory in Normandy, and when the wind was in the wrong direction the townsfolk would wrinkle their noses and complain that Dior smelled strong today. Since the financial collapse at the beginning of the Depression of his art gallery, where he had tried to sell pictures by Georges Braque, Pablo Picasso, Jean Cocteau, and Max Jacob, Christian had been quietly working for the house of Robert Piguet, attracting little attention. The whole Parisian fashion industry had collaborated during the war, and Piguet was no exception. The Nazis had tried to move "Paris" to Berlin but failed; it was too dependent on thousands of craftspeople and small ateliers, specialists in beading, feathers, and embroidery. The skills of the specialists existed in Paris and nowhere else. This was what made French fashion French and English fashion merely tailoring. (While in Germany, Hugo Boss had joined the Nazi party in 1933 and won the contract to design and supply the uniforms of the SS. Another type of tailoring.)

The winter of 1946–47 was bitter beyond belief, the coldest of the century. Siberian winds blew in across Europe. In Milan two men froze to death and the Strait of Dover recorded the lowest temperatures on the Continent. Wrapped in furs to cover their meager, government-approved "Austerity" suits and dresses purchased with clothing ration coupons, British fashion editors sat on their gilt chairs and watched not just a total change in the silhouette, but a completely new *idea* of what to wear. At the end of the show, Carmel Snow, the elderly editor of *Harper's Bazaar*, pronounced it as "a whole new look." And that was that. The imperium had spoken.

Five days later, the novelist Nancy Mitford, who had sat out the war in Paris in order to be with her French lover, would write to her sister, Diana Mosley (who had sat hers out in Holloway Prison as the loyal wife of the British fascist Oswald Mosley), that her life had been made a desert of gloom, for now all her clothes had been rendered, at a stroke, unwearable. Customers at Dior, she wrote, were fighting over them, and it was like a scene at a bargain basement sale just trying to place an order.

In that first collection, viewed by the women trying to cover their knees with their thin tweed skirts, was the "Bar" suit which I finally saw, in, so to speak, the flesh at the V&A exhibition sixty years later: an off-white shantung silk jacket with sloping shoulders and ballerina-length pleated black skirt, an outfit which requires a twenty-one-inch waist and very severe, rib-deforming corsetry, as depicted in an accompanying short film at the exhibition. Nevertheless, I appreciated its qualities as I might a painting by Leonardo da Vinci. I know now that the effortless elegance of the ensemble, as my mother would have called it, including the inverted saucer-shaped straw hat and the black gloves, the white pointed-toe shoes which look as if they are already dying to grow up and become the as-yet-to-be-invented stilettos (Roger Vivier, Dior's shoe guy, would later create those by installing a metal rod in the heel), is a masterpiece of engineering.

The illustration which would appear in French *Vogue* showed "Bar" as an airy creation, almost ethereal. In real life the wearer was held in place by a series of agonizing restraints. "Bar" is not so much sewn as constructed, using, Dior confided, "solid fabrics whose weight was reinforced with taffeta or cambric linings," not to mention underpinnings in the form of underwired bustiers, girdles, tulle and horsehair petticoats, and a strap-on device called a peplum that padded the hips in order to draw attention to the waist.

Sheer torture, but I don't care. It is the most elemental, iconic, feminine garment of the twentieth century. Whether the pleasure in wearing it overrode the pain of wearing it is a question I will return to later.

⟨⟩

A small but bestselling book, published in 1958, called *Mrs. 'Arris Goes to Paris* (or *Flowers for Mrs Harris* in the British edition) by Paul Gallico, an American author who settled in Britain before the war, describes the journey made by a widowed London cleaning lady in late middle age who, having seen a Dior couture dress in the wardrobe of one of her clients' houses, determines that, however preposterous and indeed financially impossible the goal, she is going to have her own Dior gown. Her heart and her soul are set on it. Already a devotee of flowers, an affordable though perishable beauty you can keep around the house whatever the furnishings, she sees for the first time what the human brain and human hand are capable of and her life is changed, as they say, forever:

> . . . as she stood before the stunning creations hanging in the wardrobe she found herself face to face with a new kind of beauty—an artificial one created by the hand of man the artist, but aimed directly and cunningly at the heart of a woman. . . . For it was one thing to encounter photographs of dresses, leafing through the slick pages of Vogue or Elle where, whether in colour or black and white, they were impersonal and as out of her world and her reach as the moon or the stars. It was quite another to come face to face with the real article to feast one's eyes upon its every clever stitch, to touch it, smell it, love it, and suddenly to become consumed with the fires of desire. . . . It was as though all she had missed in life through the poverty, the circumstances of her birth and class in life could be made up by becoming the holder of this one bit of feminine finery.

A combination of a moderate win on the football pools and severe scrimping and saving eventually gets her on a plane to Paris and the avenue Montaigne with £450, mainly in U.S. dollars to get around the currency regulations, bundled into her imitation crocodile handbag. She enters the salon of Christian Dior, "almost driven back by the powerful smell of elegance that assailed her once she was inside . . . compounded of perfume and fur and satins, silks and leather, jewellery and face powder. . . . It was the odour of the rich, and it made her tremble. . . ."

After numerous setbacks, such as lack of an appointment, the snobbishness of the salon manageress, and no additional currency for customs duties in those days before credit cards, Mrs. Harris eventually acquires her dress, which is called "Temptation," a black velvet floor-length gown with a jet-beaded skirt to give it weight and movement, and a cream, pink, and white chiffon, tulle, and lace top. Trying it on in the changing room, she enters the secret world of women, "the battlefield where the struggle against the ravages of age was carried on with the weapons of the dressmaker's art and where fortunes were spent in a single afternoon."

At the end of a glorious week in Paris, where, like a fairy godmother, she somehow manages to transform the fortunes of everyone she meets, including the glacial manageress and the mannequin who modeled the dress, she returns to London and immediately lends "Temptation" to someone else because she understands that the "likes of her" can never actually *wear* such a dress (where to?). The point is to have it. She needs to know it is in her wardrobe, that she can look at it whenever she wants. Above all, she needs to know that she, Mrs. Harris, is the owner of a Dior dress, when a Dior dress was the very pinnacle, the Mount Everest, the Nobel Prize of dresses.

But why does she have to have a Dior dress?

The answer to this question may be more metaphysical than psychological. It might even be existential, relating to the very essence of Mrs. Harris's being alive, breathing, existing. She could feel it impossible to live without that dress. Or that having lived fifty-eight years without it, she understands, for the first time, that she's been not fully herself. Flowers were merely the expression of a deeper longing.

At the end of the book, Gallico makes the dress not matter; it was the trip to Paris and the people she met there who counted. She's back where she started, with a damaged dress she can't wear and a room full of florists' bouquets. The novel's real lesson is of the human friendships she has made in Paris, the city "that had bestowed upon her such a priceless memory, treasure of understanding, friendship and humanity."

Fair enough, but the rest of us are still taking pleasure from looking in the window, not having staked our very beings on owning couture.

In his autobiography, published the year of his untimely death, aged only fifty-three, and a single decade after he launched the New Look, Christian Dior explained why, in his view, his first show was such a sensation. To those of us not yet born at that time, the New Look does not seem new at all. Chanel—*she* had invented a new look, had invented modern dress, but Dior's ballerina-length, romantic skirts, narrow shoulders, and teeny waists had been around for centuries; in fact Jeanne Lanvin had been making dresses similar to these in the 1920s for those of her customers who, like her middle-aged self, did not have the hipless trunks to support the tubular shape of the flapper dress.

What was new about the New Look was not new in the sense of modern, it was new in the sense that it was reviving a sensation that had been long suppressed in wartime: pleasure for the sake of it. Dior writes:

A golden age seemed to have come again. War had passed out of sight and there were no other wars on the horizon. What did the weight of my sumptuous materials, my heavy velvets and brocades, matter? When hearts were light, mere fabrics could not weigh the body down. Abundance was still too much of a novelty for a poverty cult to develop out of inverted snobbism. . . . My first creations were called names like "Love," "Tenderness,"

and "Happiness." Women have instinctively understood that I dream of
making them not only more beautiful, but also happier. That is why they
have rewarded me with their patronage.

The extraordinary privations of the Second World War for European
women have been largely forgotten. A Cecil Beaton photograph which
appeared in the September 1941 issue of *Vogue* shows a woman in
a Digby Morton suit and matching clutch turning as she passes the
bombed-out rubble of a church, the tablet with the date of its conse-
cration, 1678, still clearly readable.

"Fashion is indestructible" was either the name of the Digby Morton suit or the caption on the photograph; it isn't quite clear.

It is easy to be stylish when the shops are stuffed full of cheap
clothes made in China, when the fashion cycle is just three weeks long.
The war forcefully democratized fashion. No one was in the fashion
vanguard, fashion had come to a kind of stop, frozen by the demands
of sensible clothes. Even the wealthiest had to dress adequately for
the nightly scramble into the air-raid shelter. A mink or sable or even
fox now had added value as a really warm coat (the antifur campaign
has pointed out that the fashion for fur has died away because of central heating). Fashionable women survived the war by wearing what
they already had or having it altered; it was the opposite of consumerism—it was "Make do and mend," a doctrine that would ingrain itself
as habit into the lives of millions of women who reached adulthood
during the war and could never, in all the long years to follow, lose the
instinct to hoard string.

Across the Channel, according to an article in British *Vogue* by
Elizabeth Hoyt, an American expatriate living there, "clothing rations
are so meagre that it is impossible to dress comfortably—or even adequately—without recourse to 'Black Markets' at enormous prices. For-
tunately I had a pre-war wardrobe and wore it to shreds."

For even in times of death and horror, you still have to wear something, and it was a great struggle for the fashionable woman to remain in vogue. The well-known fallbacks of leg paint, to simulate the appearance of nylons with a wonkily drawn seam, and the wedge heel made of cork, introduced to substitute for wood and leather; the punitive British clothing rations; and the Utility styles with their skimpy skirts continuing years after the war ended—all these were forms of restraint in dress imposed by external circumstances. Wartime home dressmaking was hampered by shortages of metal to make pins, needles, and scissors. British women were driven mad by the policy of their government to restrict imports of the perm lotion "cold wave" on the wartime convoy ships from Canada. My father, who had acquired the chemical formula for "cold wave" in New York in the 1920s, and had the black market connections to get the supply of chemicals, established his profitable business as a hairdressers' supplier during the war on the back of his own product, "Barrie Cold Wave." (In desperate times, women used beets and other plants from the garden to concoct a hair dye.)

But at no point were women told that they should forget about clothes and makeup because there was a war on. Despite the difficulty of obtaining lipsticks, the painted mouth was known as the "red badge of courage": it was a defiance of war. The famous poster of the ATS warden reapplying her lipstick in the blitz was one of the iconic images of the Second World War: it said that fashion and beauty transcended death and horror, rather than being trivial and irrelevant. The government understood that fashion and beauty were the way women cheered themselves up and that without this fundamental pleasure, and the pleasure soldiers, sailors, and airmen got from looking at them, morale would sink. Trying to put together a fashionable outfit and make up your face was part of the war effort.

Joan Burstein, who would, in the early seventies, start the South Molton Street boutique Browns (having already given the teenage Manolo Blahnik his first job in the jeans department of an earlier shop), had relied on her two aunts, court dressmakers, to knock out something for her to wear during the war, using leftovers of other fabrics. The styles were copied from American magazines and what she saw at the movies. She saved her clothing coupons to buy little cotton dresses from Horrocks. But you did not feel deprived, she says. The lack made you more innovative.

"Clothes and fashion were all part of the feel-good factor," she told me. She was, at eighty-one, wearing Marni and carrying a Fendi handbag. "Even the air-raid wardens would push up a sleeve or put a shirt collar over their jacket. It was a pleasure to make yourself look good and a lot of women had to make an extra effort because their husband or boyfriend was coming home on leave. That's the *strength* of a woman."

Women thought of clothes, hair, and makeup a great deal during the war, and they thought about them whether they were breaking the Enigma code at Bletchley; working on the production lines of munitions factories making bombs, their hair pinned back from their faces under net snoods; fleeing from Paris to the comparative safety of the unoccupied south of France; or caged in the Warsaw Ghetto before its liquidation.

The French couturier Madame Grès found herself exiled in a remote village, fashioning makeshift dress forms out of hay, tin, and wood. The Comtesse de Mauduit, an American who had hidden Allied airmen in her Brittany château, was denounced by her maid and deported to the Ravensbruck concentration camp. Returning to Paris after the liberation, she arrived still in her striped uniform but looking oddly elegant, for she had come across another inmate in the camp, a forewoman from the prewar house of Schiaparelli, who had remodeled the striped suit for her.

Agnès Humbert was an art historian in her midforties when the war started, and she and her colleagues at the Musée de l'Homme in Paris quickly formed a Resistance group. Almost immediately the circle was betrayed and arrested, and Humbert was imprisoned in a

series of terrifying confinements, including months in a room little
larger than a coffin with no human contact. She describes her fellow
female prisoners in the communal cell in the Prison de la Santé as
like "a harem without a sultan. We tried out new hairstyles, did each
others' make-up, altered each others' dresses, read, told stories and
swapped recipes."

Later, transported to Germany to become slave laborers, the
female slaves were marched through the streets, where they passed
a dress shop:

> It has a large mirror, and I catch sight of myself in it. That old crone, limp-
> ing along in her preposterous clumping shoes and with her hair scraped
> into such grotesque style—that old crone is me. I have to raise my right
> hand to convince myself that the reflection in the mirror is really me. . . .
> Other women, ladies on the pavements, are wearing pretty dresses with an
> air of spring about them. This feeling like sadness that rises in my throat,
> choking me, is just absurd. Why should we blush at being paraded through
> the streets of Krefeld like this?

After the liberation, Humbert teamed up with an American officer,
trying to help alleviate the suffering of those who had managed to survive the slave labor units and deliver justice to their tormentors who
were attempting to melt back into the population. She understood that
they would not exchange addresses, they wouldn't meet up in Paris:

> . . . in Paris I wear make-up and dresses and colour my hair. Here I am
> au naturel, got up in an old pair of trousers and a factory overseer's jacket
> on which I have sewn the French flag. . . . It was war, and we were on the
> front line.

Meanwhile, in June 1945 in Berlin, a month after the mass rape of
thousands of German women by advancing soldiers of the Red Army,
the anonymous author of the diaries of those horrific events later to be

published as *A Woman in Berlin*, wrote of sitting down with a friend to sketch out the first number of a postwar women's magazine and think up a name for it. It would definitely, she writes, contain the word *new*.

The following day, June 9, 1945, she walked twelve miles to find nettles to eat to supplement her rations of groats and sugar. In the afternoon she visited the hairdresser "for the first time in ages." Photographs of the bombed Berlin show a city aerially destroyed. Ruins. Broken glass. Dust. The timber of fallen trees lie along the streets like felled stone columns. The devastation seems as old as Pompey.

Somehow the owner of the salon managed to salvage one mirror and one halfway serviceable hair dryer. He washed "about a pound of dirt" out of her hair. With a hairdo, the raped and vanquished are, she writes, at least to themselves, more than "rubble-women and trash."

The previous month in Lower Saxony, Lieutenant Colonel Mervin Willett Gonin, one of the first British soldiers to liberate Bergen-Belsen, wrote the following entry in his diary.

> *I can give no adequate description of the Horror Camp in which my men and myself were to spend the next month of our lives. . . . It was shortly after the [British Red Cross] arrived, though it may have no connection, that a very large quantity of lipstick arrived. This was not at all what we men wanted. We were screaming for hundreds and thousands of other things and I don't know who asked for lipstick. I wish so much that I could discover who did it. It was the action of genius, sheer unadulterated brilliance. I believe nothing did more for these internees than the lipstick. . . . At last someone had done something to make them individuals again: they were someone, no longer merely the number tattooed on the arm. At last they could take an interest in their appearance. That lipstick started to give them back their humanity.*

It is quite horrible to think of those bald, shivering, emaciated women, covered in sores and lice, gruesomely decorated with a slash of red across their mouths, but for them that wasn't the point. How they looked in the mirror, which they would not have had access to, was less important than the knowledge that lipstick was the attribute of a woman, not that word the Nazis used for them: *Stücke*, or pieces.

The defeated women of Berlin, the liberated women of Bergen-Belsen and of the French Resistance all had in common this collective desire to look pretty. It survived intact, when the rest of their humanity had been assaulted almost beyond repair. I cannot see how such an instinct could be described as superficial if it can withstand the almost total destruction of the personality.

∽

In Britain, postwar austerity bit even harder than it had during the war. The U.S. government's Marshall Plan, rescuing Germany from destitution and rebuilding it as a democracy, did not extend to Britain, which was still paying back wartime loans and enduring rationing well into the 1950s. The New Look, the epitome of the pleasure principle, required a radical alteration in the shape of a woman's body. The tiny waist and wide hips could only be achieved by "foundation garments," but corsetry, regarded as inessential, was still banned under rationing "except on doctor's orders."

The essence of the New Look was frivolity, pleasure, wastefulness. It was resoundingly nonutilitarian. The British government's response to the New Look was to try to deny that it even existed. Alison Settle, editor of *Vogue*, was forbidden by the Board of Trade, under its president, the future prime minister, Harold Wilson, even to mention Dior in her pages. The need for income from exports restricted the textiles available for home consumption and the Board believed that the New Look would create impossible demands for additional fabric. Wilson told fashionable women that if they wanted fuller skirts, they would have to have fewer skirts. Even in America, there was public disapproval among patriotic women and when Dior himself toured the U.S. to promote his collection, he was greeted by crowds of women protesting against the new, wasteful skirt lengths, the dresses literally being torn by indignant matrons from the padded hips of the models.

But of course there were always exceptions. At a secret session held at the British embassy in Paris, Princess Margaret was shown the New Look. The dress demand of the two young princesses, constantly in the public eye, and the need for society clothes for state events stimulated Britain's own fashion industry. The Royal College of Art opened its first fashion department, inspired by the New Look, and designers such as Norman Hartnell, Hardy Amies, Digby Morton, and Edward Molyneux brought the traditions of British tailoring to the exacting demands of couture.

At the end of the war, the hunger for pleasure was so profound that only high-minded ascetics could turn their noses up at new clothes. A new dress. What did it mean for those women who had endured and survived mass warfare? A private client of the house of Balmain wrote, in a thank-you note on receipt of her new dress:

> It gave me a taste for life again. Never mind the dress: its sheer arrival was enough, carried by a man in a uniform, in its enormous new cardboard box, surrounded by pounds of tissue paper. When I signed for it I felt everything was worth while, that life was exciting again. Thank you. . . .

Hardly anyone can own couture, but anyone can own a blurry, approximate copy of the basic *idea* of such a garment. The New Look was copied by industrial methods, on an industrial scale. Everyone wanted cheap up-to-the-minute stuff.

To Joan Burstein, seeing the New Look for the first time as a twenty-year-old, the sensation was . . . it was . . . "It was like, ah!" And she let out a long breath. "Something extraordinary and wonderful had happened because it was so extravagant. It was like a release for women. No more restrictions, and it was beautiful and it was new and it was different. A tightly fitted little jacket and a volume of skirt for daywear—nobody has ever been able to re-create that.

"It was unbelievably exciting. Suddenly this man had created beautiful women again, not women living under a cloud. That was what he managed to express, and even if she was under a cloud, wearing these clothes managed to transform their lives. Dior had a statement. What did Yves Saint Laurent have? A trench coat."

Dior was asked repeatedly why his New Look was such a sensation. He referred to the crazy times just before the war: Schiaparelli with her hats like lobsters and the *zazou* craze of Paris during the war—wide shoulders; short, pleated skirts; striped stockings; and shoes with thick wooden soles, a bohemian's thumbs-down to the Nazis.

"I believe it was due to the fact that I brought back the neglected art of pleasing," he modestly said.

Out of suffering comes the demand for pleasure. When we have suffered we do not care less about clothes but more. To love clothes is to embrace life in all its joyous variety, even if all you ever do is turn the pages of a magazine and long for fairyland, crave couture ballgowns you will never own. We all need daydreams. One lipstick alone can go a long, long way.

·⁀·

And this brings me to Catherine Hill, whose story throws a strong light onto one of the darkest places of the twentieth century, proving beyond a doubt that even in the valley of the shadow of death the human heart can long for a hat.

CATHERINE HILL: *NEVER WEAR BLACK*

I WOULD NOT describe Catherine Hill as an elegant woman because I think of elegance as being composed of two parts chic and one part aloofness. To be elegant is a discipline of the body, the refinement of form acquired by natural instinct and study. An elegant woman is always slightly apart; her clothes seem wary of any disturbance to the harmony of the effect, however effortlessly they appear to be arranged on the body. The elegant woman is to be admired; but to be desired requires a certain untidiness and disorder, if only in the form of a carelessly undone button.

Catherine is not cool, she is hot. Apart from some jeans and a Dior bag, there is not, as far as I can tell, a single item of black in her enormous walk-in closet. Nor among the rows of shoes, all the Roger Viviers, the Manolo Blahniks, the Jimmy Choos. Her hair is platinum blond.

She rises every morning, not too early, dresses, and walks across her Toronto street to Starbucks, where she has coffee. It's a fashion neighborhood and a fashion street, and the young things come and go in their Chloé and their Louboutins.

Catherine Hill, who will not state her age, is wearing one of her collection of Christian Lacroix jackets, or maybe today it's the John Galliano denim jacket with the asymmetrical mink collar; a white and gold Armani T-shirt above her boot-cut jeans ("They're not designer, I bought them at a young person's shop"); a long chain looped from her waist like the rappers; high-heeled Roger Vivier gold shoes; and a mulberry leather Dior handbag. After drinking her latte, she carefully reapplies her coral lipstick in the mirror of a gold Guerlain powder compact.

She is not so much the sum of what she wears but how she commands her whole appearance, this provocation. If I could situate her anywhere and show her to you, it would be drinking a cocktail or a glass of champagne in the shade of the palm trees that grow in the gardens of the late Gianni Versace's mansion in Miami Beach. A spot located somewhere between the old and the new worlds. Punk luxe, but always in color.

After coffee we go back across the street, to her large apartment above Hazelton Lanes, a mall of high-end fashion stores, where, until quite recently, she had a store herself.

She is going to tell me about her life in fashion, about the importance of what we wear, why it matters. My reason for crossing the Atlantic at my own expense to meet her is that I have a sense that she *is* fashion, but not in a way that fashion's critics would understand the term.

Catherine begins to talk first of painful, recent things, then of her childhood before the war. "No matter at what stage of life I am and what is happening, there is always a link to the past," she tells me. "I feel that I am special and I am different because I am a Holocaust survivor. I'm so lucky to survive because there's something to show for it. It has nothing to do with success, it's life—the survival of life and the continuity of that life, how precious it is."

◦◦◦

She arrived in Canada as a refugee a few years after the end of the Second World War, all alone, without parents or brothers and sisters, uncles or aunts. Her mother had not survived the selections at Auschwitz-Birkenau, her father died of typhus in the camp. After the liberation, her bones rattling, Catherine had tried returning home, to the town where she was born, whose status and nationality changed from month to month according to the whims of the war-ring powers. Strangers had opened the door of her family's apart-ment and told her she had no home anymore. Her only surviving relative was a cousin.

Meeting up with another survivor, she traveled to Rome, where she was classified as a Displaced Person, stateless, and like all the refu-gees, she had been waiting. Waiting to be told where to go, waiting for the quotas. The Allied powers were in no hurry to take in the refugees. Each country imposed its own restrictions on the numbers they would admit. Catherine was under the care of the Joint, the American Jew-ish Joint Distribution Committee, which had come to Europe to help process the refugees and find homes for them.

If it had been her choice, she would have stayed in Rome, for there everything was, she remembers, "so maximum"—how the women dressed, how the stores looked, and the gourmet food. Rome had given Catherine back the joy of life after all the horror, the pain, the annihilating loneliness.

In a year or so, learning how to be free and not a slave laborer, how to eat and dress and feel, she was offered the choice of a new country—Australia or Canada. Canada, she said, because it was part of America—well, that's the way it looks on the map. The Canadian government was making the refugees an offer: in exchange for a nationality, they had to serve out a one-year contract. Either she could be a nanny in a private home or work in a hospital. She tried both.

She made her first landfall in North America in the middle of win-ter in a city called Halifax, Nova Scotia, in the distant Maritime Prov-inces, stepping into a country gray and full of snow, wearing a little green coat and little green sandals. She did not really understand where she was. Was this America or not? From Halifax, they took her to Montreal, which suited her because she spoke French and did not speak English (it is her seventh language).

In Quebec she consoled herself with film and fashion magazines, and reading them, began to learn a little English. By now she was acquiring a wardrobe: a pair of shoes, some blouses, and after she had fulfilled her contract she thought she might do some modeling.

She was the in-store mannequin at a little dress shop for a while; they didn't pay much so she took a course at the Fashion Arts Academy where she learned for the first time exactly how a dress was made and won a prize: "I got a little bit of taste and knowledge, and when I was looking for jobs, that's when I found an ad that my future husband put in which said they were looking for women with imagination and fashion direction, not knowing he would marry me."

For most of the 1950s Catherine was a middle-class Montreal housewife and mother. She prefers not to talk about her husband and why the marriage did not work out. He was a good man, he was kind, she says, but on the issue of understanding survivors, like many others, he failed.

It was as a married woman that Catherine first began to develop her understanding of clothes and fashion. "I realized what clothes do, how they make you feel, and that was the beginning, when I really felt some connection with clothes. Suddenly I felt the desire not only to have the enjoyment of constantly wearing these beautiful things but also, looking around, I started to observe how people dressed, and I could begin to tell why this didn't look good on a woman and I became a little bit critical."

She was at liberty to re-create the life she had seen in Rome, the expansive luxury of those with money to spend on clothes and food. She embraced all the possibilities of living in the fifties, that affluent decade. She went shopping.

In 1955 Catherine gave birth to her daughter, her only child, Stefani, named after her own late father, Stefan. By the beginning of the 1960s, the marriage was drawing to an end. She had a friend, the deliciously named Lou-Lou-Belle, an interior designer who also worked in the gift department of Eaton's, the Canadian department store chain. They had lunch one day and talked about Catherine's imminent separation and Lou-Lou-Belle suggested she find a job.

What could she do? She was trained for nothing, but Lou-Lou-Belle said: "Catherine, you have such tremendous taste and you just look like fashion all the time. You should think of going into the fashion business." And then Lou-Lou-Belle arranged an appointment for her friend at Eaton's.

Catherine had no idea how to dress to apply for a job at a department store. She put on her jewels. She was interviewed by the merchandising manager, who was French, and said she looked too rich to work. The job didn't pay much, only around $60 a week. It was not, she thought, a great beginning, but it was something, and the something was freedom. Catherine wanted independence, not alimony. "I have a thing about lawyers," she says. "I don't like to litigate and yet somehow I still want justice, so I decided that if I didn't need anybody's money, I just wanted my liberty and freedom. That job I took was one of the best decisions I made for my career because that was the beginning of the fashion thing."

The work was more physically hard than she had imagined. "Every night I had to come home and soak my feet in Epsom salts. You couldn't sit down; it was a very, very difficult job. Most of the saleswomen were in their sixties; they wore low-heeled shoes and I wore high-heeled shoes, the clothes from my marriage. I was very tired, it was exhausting; you had to be there from nine o'clock until six o'clock, and then I would go home and look after my daughter and do the cooking. It was a difficult period."

Despite the physical exhaustion, it was these early years at Eaton's that gave Catherine an opportunity to appraise the merchandise and to develop an understanding of the enormous deficiencies of the women's wear on offer in one of Canada's great cities in the early 1960s. There were cheap dresses for older women, American clothes, and a few European lines. Canadian clothes were made by Canadian companies and lacked the quality and panache of what she had seen in Europe.

"I realized that the tremendous difference between Europeans and Canadians was that the Canadians always came in and looked for clothes for a special occasion, whereas in Europe a woman gets up, gets dressed, goes for lunch."

Holt Renfrew was the store for the carriage trade—the upscale shoppers—and Eaton's was trying in a small way to compete for a share of its market. Catherine studied the stock. She learned to distinguish between good and bad. In Rome she had seen "a tremendous amount of clothes" and had been a keen reader of fashion magazines. One of the buyers had been born in Paris and had acquired for the store a collection of what was then called sportswear, which really meant the death-knell of the fifties look and the beginning of casual separates: tops and bottoms which did not necessarily match and which could be worn without formal accessories like a hat or gloves. To put together a chic look in sportswear was the newest thing and no one was entirely sure how it was done.

Perhaps Catherine would have left Eaton's and found something better to do with her talents than sell dresses for weddings and bar mitzvahs to provincial women were it not for a customer who arrived one day on her floor with a request that she find something nice as a present for his wife.

Catherine had always spoken her mind; even in childhood she had a habit of speaking the truth, the words already out of her mouth before she considered the consequences. She remembered how she was the only girl in her class at school who admitted to the teacher that she had not done the homework for a lesson and so could not be expected to know the answer. Her tongue got her into trouble, but would sometimes surprise and disarm the people she met.

"He was very well dressed, an elderly gentleman. I looked at him and I said to myself, So what do you want, a scarf? I said, 'If you're looking for a gift for your wife, I think maybe you should go to another store, because in this section I can't think of anything.' "

The next day she was called into the office of the merchandising manager. "You know, you talk too much," he said to her. "Yesterday you were talking to a gentleman and you criticized the store, and you said that the merchandise is not good, and the buying is no good. You know who you were talking to? That's Jack Eaton, the owner of the store."

"I started to cry because I knew I was going to be fired any minute. He said, 'You're such a big mouth.' I was still crying; he gave me his handkerchief from his pocket." Jack Eaton, he told her, was sending her back to Europe.

He sent her back as a buyer, with a budget of a quarter of a million dollars. It's a fairy tale, but fairy tales do, of course, happen from time to time. He was trying to compete with Holt Renfrew and something was wrong with his stock. If there was nothing good enough for his wife, there was nothing he could sell to the other wealthy women of Montreal.

Her first stop was London. Eaton's had offices in every major fashion city but Catherine turned up and told them they were buying all the wrong things. It was difficult and stressful to be so at odds with the people who should have been on her side, but the Eaton's buyers did not understand what was happening in fashion in the early 1960s.

"I decided I was going to stand firm and I was going to find these new designers, so everything I bought for the store was totally different from what the buyers had bought before. The English designers I bought at that time were Frank Usher, Jean Muir. All I know is when it came in and we put it on the floor, not only did we have to reorganize, but we had to get new people to sell these clothes, we had to get some younger people."

Catherine's innovative buying in Europe resulted in a stand-alone, in-store boutique being created for her, the New Orleans Boutique, which eventually went into every Eaton's across the country. From New York she was buying Bill Blass and Anne Klein. "I had such a reputation, I refused to buy copies. In Montreal there was a group of manufacturers; they were producing wonderful clothes, but what they did, they went to Europe and they copied. I refused. I said, 'I'm not going to mix these things in, I'm going to buy European and American clothes,' and so they got very upset. I created a certain atmosphere there, but the bottom line was that my buying made money."

She considers her years at Eaton's in the 1960s as a kind of laboratory of revolutionary ideas. In New York, Paris, London, Milan, she would go from showroom to showroom looking for clothes that not only had good taste, but a combination of pieces that was different from what anybody else in Canada did. "I just bought what I liked and what I thought made sense for me and for the city. It was an exciting period, a learning period. I had this beautiful shop in the middle of the third floor and I was the competition with the guy who had the major designers from Paris, I had to do things in a lesser price but emulate what he did."

Throughout the 1960s Catherine was being headhunted by other stores. By the end of the decade she was asked to come to Toronto to take over as fashion director at Creeds, the fashion store. It was not just the money and the status that influenced her decision to move, but what her parents back in Europe during the war had lacked: a heightened sense of danger, and the instinct of self-preservation which tells you to get out while you can.

During that decade a Marxist separatist organization, the Front de Libération du Québec, had been carrying out a series of terrorist acts. In early 1969 they bombed the Montreal stock exchange; later in the year they attacked the house of the city's mayor. In 1970 they kidnapped and subsequently murdered a leading politician, Pierre Laporte.

"I felt that I wanted to move away from Montreal. I saw some danger. The pivot was really this killing, and that there was going to be a war, and I thought, I'm not going to wait for it, I'm going to be smarter this time and I'm going to avoid it. I was asked to be the fashion director of Creeds and he had Herve Leger, Zandra Rhodes, designers that I was not able to do in Eaton's, so I had the opportunity to go to Europe to buy, and I said, okay, I'm going to do it." She moved with her daughter to Toronto.

In Florence she saw Missoni, a brand which Diana Vreeland had brought to America with the famous declaration "There are not just colors, there are also tones." In their showroom Catherine fell in love with the zigzag patterns, the proliferation of colors, the intellectual design. No one in Canada stocked Missoni, which had only recently been written up in the U.S. by *Women's Wear Daily*. She told her boss she had to buy the line. They went to Harry's Bar for lunch that day and he told her that Missoni would never sell, it was too quirky, too artistic.

"I'd brought fake furs in from New York, we went to buy Lanvin in Paris, but everything I did, he was so insecure and taken aback. Nobody knew what hit them; they could not understand the mix. It should have really worked. He lost his confidence in me. They did stupid things. I brought in a dress, let's say it was three thousand dollars or four thousand, and one of the assistants decides he's going to give it to a manufacturer in Toronto and they're going to make a hundred copies and they're going to put it next to the dress and sell it for $200 to $300. I said, 'Eddie, you can't do this, you're killing your own trade.' But the staff were worried about their jobs."

"The taste of Canadian women in the sixties and seventies was very conservative. Missoni when it first appeared was really sportswear, but it was very colorful and today it's nothing revolutionary, but for them to understand it, there was art in it. I always feel the most important thing in clothing is repetition of something that was there before, but introducing it in a new way, in a new format, I never seen it before. So I looked for innovative things. I had been seven years at Eaton's. I was exposed to a merchandising system and the politics of buyers, how they always bought the navy suit because they saw twenty of them last year. They never went out on a limb because they were worried about their jobs, about what's going to sell. They did the same thing every day and they didn't have the free spirit or the desire to be innovative."

One day after two years with the company her boss fired her. He told her she did not have the talent for buying.

It was the most devastating blow, this rejection, reducing her to a zero.

"I just wanted to make the life that I was given after the war worth-while every minute of the day. The meaning of life is different for the people like me who went to Auschwitz. We're chasing the rainbow, looking for joy and some sort of happiness. I was in this city, I had a wonderful penthouse place, I had my daughter. Then I lost my job. Everything abrupt that happens is so painful and so traumatic, but it happens because it catapults me to something else. There was a pattern set, and I really have nothing to do with it, the abrupt thing—it says, 'I don't care however hard you try, you have to do something else, and there's nothing you can do about it.' "

So her second child was born, her shop, Chez Catherine.

Especially designed gas protection costumes at a reasonable price of £40. This outfit is made of pure oiled silk and is available in dawn, apricot, rose, amethyst, Eau de Nil green and pastel pink. The wearer can cover a distance of two hundred yards through mustard gas and the suit can be slipped over ordinary clothes in thirty-five seconds. A special pair of mittens is supplied while the hood top is designed to cover up the head space unprotected by the ordinary gas mask.

∽ Harvey Nichols advertisement, 1939

TO THE SHOPS

MY MOTHER, WHO died at the age of eighty-one from a condition called vascular dementia, could not remember the beginning of a short sentence by the time she was approaching its conclusion, which more or less eliminated from her diminishing world the pleasures of conversation. In the last weeks of her life the part of her brain which controlled language began to malfunction and she started to speak in weird phrases, which, if you listened to them carefully enough, were made up of words and syllables from both English and Yiddish, her first language, which during the long years of her illness she appeared to have completely forgotten.

Her last full, coherent, grammatically intact message to the world was uttered to my sister: "I like your earrings." Her last words to me as mother to daughter, the person she knew to be her daughter, and not merely someone she knew she knew, had been stated a few months earlier: "I don't like your hair."

But before she became immobilized by incontinence and other terrible afflictions, the one activity my mother was still capable of participating in heart and soul, with a fully functioning mind, was shopping for clothes. She would wander along the street crying and moaning, me gripping her arm for fear she would fall into the traffic. Her own fate was terrible to her, and she knew it. Then we would get to the small clothing section of the Upper Street branch of Marks & Spencer and her identity re-formed; she was a human being once again, capable of assessing the quality of knits and whether this season's hemlines were flattering on her small frame. The shopper's soul shout, *"I want!"* raced through her bloodstream. Once, I pointed out that Marks & Spencer had introduced a delivery service for certain postcodes. "Oh, yeah?" she said. "And you'll pay through the nose for it." But a second or two later, she was grasping my arm and asking had I seen the sign which announced that Marks & Spencer now delivered to certain postcodes.

I took her to buy an outfit for my sister's wedding. As soon as she had ascended the escalator she seized on a Ralph Lauren skirt and Jaeger blouse. She scurried around the store holding fabrics together, "because I've got to match the navy." She cried and stamped her foot when the blouse was too big in the collar, revealing her ruined neck. I understood for the first time that she always wore a little scarf not because her old bones were cold, but because she understood the feminine art of concealment, how to cover and flatter. She had no intention of being mutton dressed as lamb.

The outfit, which I paid for, cost a bomb. In the taxi back to the home where my sister and I had incarcerated her against her will when she was considered no longer able to function alone, she held her shopping bags with a radiant face, looked at me, eyes milky with innocence and bewilderment. "How are we related?" she asked.

I believe that when the brain is ravaged by illness, certain sectors of it, which correspond to the core of one's being, one's very self, one's soul, if you like, are preserved intact. A man who mistakes his wife for a hat, according to Oliver Sacks, may still be able to sit down at the piano and play a concerto. Shopping was what my mother had always excelled at, it was her deepest and most enduring interest. Eventually it was how she knew she was alive, not immolated in a terrifying twilight of incomprehension, each moment suspended alone from the one that had preceded it. Life was the perpetual present tense from which she struggled and usually failed to escape. Time was a prison. Only clothes and shopping could liberate her from this hell; medical science had nothing at all to offer. When she shopped, and when she looked in the wardrobe in the morning to choose her day's outfit, she was temporarily herself.

She had grown up during the Depression, married after the war. Was a young matron in the fifties, that decade of abundance and pleasure, of mink stoles and pearl necklaces and diamond clips and beautiful handbags made in Italy. Outside my bedroom, on a shelf, is a row of her beautiful bags.

Some years ago, the daughter of a famous feminist told me that her mother had been a difficult woman, but that she respected her for her stand against injustice, for her fierce moral code, and that these were the enduring lessons she had learned from her. She asked me what I had learned from my mother, and thinking for a moment, I came up with the phrase which had etched itself on my childhood: "A good handbag makes the outfit." We put it in my mother's death notice in the *Jewish Chronicle* when she died:

> *After a long illness bravely borne. She taught us to respect others, that chicken soup can cure almost everything and a good handbag makes the outfit.*

My mother's absorption in shopping began in the early part of her life and, it should be obvious if you've read this far, it is the inheritance her two daughters received from her. She imprinted upon us the notion that shopping was a serious activity, not to be taken lightly, requiring stamina and acquired skills. It was not by any means to be regarded as an adjunct of housekeeping. It was almost a career in and of itself, for to have the right clothes and the right furnishings in the suburbs meant that you needed to know what you were doing.

Like my father's parents, my maternal grandparents had arrived in England at the turn of the century from the environs of Kiev in the Ukraine. Both died before I was born, so I never knew them. I was brought up to believe that my grandfather was a cobbler, but the truth was somewhat more modest and more shocking: he went from house to house buying the shoes of people who had recently died, then refurbishing them, and my grandmother sold them in a stall at Bootle market. Out of such enterprise Simon Marks built Marks & Spencer, but nobody in my mother's family struck it rich. They all went into the needle trades, apart from one brother who became a cabinetmaker.

The youngest of six children, my mother's older brothers and sisters were already out at work and earning wages while she was at school, and she would later be described by her siblings as a "spoilt child." She had what they had not, shoes, for example. For footwear was considered something one only wore for best, lest the expensive leather wear out.

Until the thirties, the working class were used to having only two sets of clothing, one for the weekday, worn literally day in and day out (including underwear), and Sunday best. The cost of clothes more fully represented their true worth then: a man's shirt could cost a week's wages. Even the middle classes had fewer suits and dresses than we do today. When the weekday outfit could no longer be patched or turned (a skill I remember some families still using in my own childhood), it would be cut down for a child; the adult got a new outfit for the Sabbath and the Sunday suit or dress became the everyday outfit. There was little demarcation between smart and casual. Men wore shirts and ties all week long.

My mother, as a teenager, would go with all her friends, a length of material under their arms, to a local dressmaker who only had one pattern, with its sole variety in the neckline (round, V, or boat—your choice), so they all turned up at the dance in essentially the same outfit. My mother wanted far better for herself, and I cannot help but believe that she would have seen about town, in and out of the shops, the figure of Emily Tinne, who was, as far as anyone knows, the world's first recorded shopaholic. For as my mother pressed her nose against the plate-glass window of Liverpool's most exclusive department store, George Henry Lee's, inside, Emily Tinne was buying.

From sometime in 1910, eight years before my mother was born, Tinne began shopping, and over a thirty-year period she set out on a journey of massive retail acquisition, with a hunger for new clothes which did not come to an end until 1940, when the government issued ration books that covered not just food but clothing. By the time the war was over she was nearly sixty, and perhaps the obsessive desire to shop had burnt out in her at last, or, more likely, the private wealth which had funded her long shopping spree had dried up.

The dresses, coats, hats, underwear, shoes, stoles, and furs Mrs. Tinne bought were more than anyone could wear in a lifetime, and they now represent the largest single museum collection of one woman's clothes, one woman's personal style, a mere fraction of which went on display at the Walker Art Gallery in Liverpool in 2005. For Mrs. Tinne, like a true shopaholic, often did not even unwrap the things she bought; they lay for half a century in the original boxes with the handwritten bill, indicating the date, price, and place she bought them.

Her family's money was based, as much of the city's wealth was, on coffee, cotton, shipping, and rum. The Tinnes owned the first motorcar in Liverpool. Emily's daughter, Dr. Alexine Tinne, told me she believed her mother began shopping because she was bored. "She was an extremely intelligent woman and she would go into town just to occupy herself," she says.

There are no great designer labels in the collection, no Poiret, Chanel, Molyneux, or even Susan Small, and this is what makes Emily Tinne's wardrobe so fascinating. For like the overwhelming majority of middle-class provincial women, she shopped mainly in local department stores. Until the 1960s, Liverpool had at least five, and Emily's evident favorites, judging by the labels, were George Henry Lee and the adjacent Bon Marché, which Lee's would take over in 1961. These stores made their own copies of the latest styles.

The puzzle about the clothes is not just that many of them remained unworn, but that they were things she had little or no occasion to wear. For the wife of a local doctor there were limited opportunities to dress up, and the Tinnes did not seem to have had a particularly active social life; the doctor held surgeries every evening and they went to few parties. Perhaps, like many middle-class families before the war, the couple dressed for dinner, but their daughter has no recollections of this. "I remember my mother in rather uninteresting black things," she says. "She wasn't very stylish and I just can't imagine her wearing some of those dresses. Her family would have been shocked."

One remarkable clue to why Emily Tinne bought so many clothes was the changing fortunes of the city itself. In 1910, when she married, Liverpool was at the height of its powers as the greatest port in the British Empire, the gateway to the colonies, with millions of tons of shipping on the Mersey bringing goods from Africa and the Americas. By the 1930s, the Depression had plunged it into poverty. Dr. Tinne, in those days before the National Health Service (NHS), was using his middle-class surgery in Aigburth to subsidize the treatment of the poor in working-class Garston. Alexine Tinne believes that her mother bought extravagant furs and evening gowns to help the shopgirls who were paid exclusively on commission. She shopped as an act of philanthropy.

As her uncontrolled shopping increased, storage became a problem. The Tinnes had moved into Clayton Lodge, a large house in the suburb of Aigburth which stood in three acres of gardens. By the 1930s, they had fewer servants, and Emily took over what had been their quarters to house the huge numbers of things she had bought. Packed away in tea chests, they were moved to the cellar during the war. After her death in 1966 at the age of eighty, Emily's daughter could no longer maintain the large house and began to address what to do about her mother's clothes. "When I opened up the cellar I was shattered at the volume of stuff and had little idea of what was in those crates," she says. "I used to put out two tea chests each week and someone from the museum would come and collect them."

Was Emily Tinne's shopaholism an illness, a psychological disorder? Or was it at the extreme end of the private passion that so many of us have for going to the shops? There is no sense, in her daughter's recollections, of her being an unhappy woman; in fact she is remembered as a warm and loving mother. She did not need and had neither the figure nor the occasion to wear a satin bias-cut backless evening gown similar to that worn by Jean Harlow in the movies. But the dress fulfilled some *want* in her. And there was no financial disincentive to buy it, and as she was aiding the impoverished shopgirls of the Depression, there was no great harm in buying it either.

I believe that Emily Tinne went shopping because she enjoyed it. It was something to do. Maybe it began as a release from boredom, as her daughter suggests, and became a habit; her husband worked long hours, she was underemployed at home with a large house and servants, but she liked shopping for its own sake, she liked being in the shops, and the act of actually paying for the goods, rather than just looking, was an incidental aspect of the experience. Perhaps it was, as her daughter suggests, a philanthropic gesture. But if she had been concerned by the plight of impoverished shopgirls in the Depression, she could have thrown herself into some form of political or charitable activity or what used to be called settlement work before it became known as social work.

Instead, she continued to do what she liked doing—shopping.

The whole experience of this activity, for my mother, as I imagine her watching Mrs. Tinne, must have seemed one of easeful rapture. You didn't even have to take the goods home on the bus, for they would be delivered direct to your house by a George Henry Lee van, along with the invoice. George Henry Lee had tearooms and a restaurant. You could order a sophisticated little lunch. You could eat an egg mayonnaise wearing a small hat with a veil.

And this is what my mother would do herself, two decades later, in the 1950s, with me schlepping along after her, though sometimes, more excitingly, we were shopping for me: taken to try on a royal blue velvet dress with real hand-stitched smocking, black patent Startrite T-bar shoes, and white ankle socks trimmed with lace. A framed, hand-colored portrait of me in this ensemble, with a bow in my artificially waved hair, stood for many years on an occasional table near the front door of our house, built in 1959 and decorated by an interior designer from Leeds who did it up in George IV–meets–Constance Spry style, all eau de Nil and gold.

My mother shopped because shopping was what she was good at. She had an unerring capacity to enter any store and pick out the most expensive item in it; she had a fantastic eye. Even though she almost never had the money to buy the best thing in the shop, she knew what the best thing was, and following that, the calculations you needed to make in order to get as close to it as possible: such as when the sales started, or where you could get really good copies, or which second-hand shops had the kind of stock she was looking for.

She had, in other words, taste. And she learned her taste from a variety of sources, such as reading magazines, listening to friends' recommendations, but above all, spending a great deal of time actually in the shops, looking at things and learning how to discern the good, the bad, and the very best. Friends queued up to go shopping with her, for they knew she would take them to the right places and make them try on the things she knew would suit them.

Poor her, running headlong into the 1960s with a daughter who deliberately frayed the hems of her jeans and wore a handbag made out of a bit of old carpet, instead of Young Jaeger.

But of course all daughters eventually turn into their mothers, and she had encoded herself inside me already. I feel her most intensely when I am walking along Bond Street early on a spring morning; around me the shops are just opening and I am wearing the right clothes, and importantly, the right scent. Clickety-clack along the echoing pavements. I am *une femme d'une certaine age*. Which is fine, because I am now of a *certain age* (the age at which others should stop being so bloody rude and asking my age).

I'm entitled. Entitled to be walking along Bond Street and entitled to go inside Hermès and inquire the length of the waiting list for a Birkin handbag ("The waiting list is closed, Madame. I can put you on the waiting list to join the waiting list"). And why not put yourself on the waiting list for something you can't afford, because the fact you are on the waiting list implies that you are the sort of person who might one day own a Birkin at a cost of £3,500 ($5,600), even though you know perfectly well that you won't?

Mounting a defense of shopping inevitably becomes an argument in favor of capitalism, and then we're into politics, and if you wanted to read about politics, rather than the human spirit and how it survives even in adversity, saying "Rejoice!" again, you'd have bought another book.

Most hostile responses to shopping see it is an act of acquisition, of avarice and greed for things that we do not need but advertising and marketing have made us think we want, a condition which Marx called "false consciousness." We are dupes, and only the strong individualist can hold out against mass consumption.

And there are others, of course, who truthfully say that they have no political objection to shopping but they just can't stand it as an activity and regard it as a waste of time.

Against whom I would set those of us who regard it as a pleasure.

What does this pleasure consist of, and why do others not experience it? Why do they feel, instead, a sense of panic, overwhelmed by what they describe as "too much choice"? Why do I like *looking* at other people's gardens, while content to allow my own to degenerate into a badly designed, overgrown jungle of strangled plants and rapacious weeds? Because I can't be bothered going out there to do the work of making it bloom. I watch the flowers wither and die from lack of water and mourn them. Opening the door and filling a watering can passes fleetingly through my mind without me actually doing anything about it. But were I to wake up and know, at the moment of the mind streaming back from dark into light and consciousness, that what a new navy linen jacket needs is a scarf with a bit of red in it, then I will have ants in my pants until I can get to the shops to find that scarf.

◌◦

Shopping. A gerund which did not exist before the middle of the eighteenth century because it did not exist in the way we understand it now. It involved the single revolutionary and emancipatory act of middle-class women with disposable incomes leaving the house. Before this, the goods, or the people who made them, came *to* the house, either the tailors and seamstresses or the peddlers who sold door-to-door to the poor. The tradition of women going shopping is not only rooted in the fact that they have always been in charge of the housekeeping, or that women have a love of finery not shared by their male counterparts. (As any costume history shows, that the bland muted palette, decoration-free surfaces, and glacierlike speed of changes in the style of menswear is a twentieth-century invention. Sixteenth-century man was covered in gold embroidery and jeweled codpieces.) When women started to shop seriously, in the nineteenth century, it was the first development in their liberation; a stage on the journey which would lead to the vote.

The first known use of the word *shopping* is recorded by the OED in

1764: "Ladies are said to go a Shoping, when, in the Forenoon, sick of themselves, they order the Coach, and driving from Shop to Shop." In Fanny Burney's novel *Evelina*, published in 1778, the eponymous heroine, newly arrived in London, writes a letter home: "We have been a-shopping, as Mrs Mirvan calls it," which indicates that the term is new to Evelina, a girl from the provinces. The earliest example of *shopping* without the preceding *a*- is recorded in Fanny Burney's journals, from 1782: "They spent at one shopping £20 in Gauzes two or three years ago!"

The shopping that Burney's female characters did was at small drapers' shops, in London, Bath, or market towns. The history of shopping as a modern activity begins in the nineteenth century, with the industrial revolution, mass manufacture, and the development of the department store, or *grand magasin*.

The railways brought people quickly into city centers. The city rose as a megalopolis, where millions lived and worked. London fanned out from its inner center; new suburbs of terraced Victorian houses accommodated the clerks, the typists, shoe salesmen, and trains connected them to their jobs. Without a city, there is no shopping as we understand it today. And without there first being a city, the suburban mall could not have come into existence. The railways built the city, cars built the mall.

There are two types of living: a living done on city pavements, where you are on display, and a living done mainly in a vehicle or an interior. Street style and car style are two different things, as the fashion in New York and the fashion in Los Angeles attest. The nineteenth century first brought women out onto the streets in huge numbers, on their way to and from work and to and from the shops. "At first," writes Elizabeth Wilson, "the women of the bourgeoisie had gone out cloaked and veiled. It was hardly respectable for a woman to be on the streets at all—and she must of course be chaperoned, or accompanied by a footman." But by the 1860s, New York women were already wearing the Fifth Avenue Walking Dress, based on the hunting jacket, as if simply parading through the newly built streets were a sporting activity, or a form of exercise like jogging which required special clothes.

In 1883 Émile Zola would publish a novel, *The Ladies' Paradise*, based on Le Bon Marché in Paris. Until 1852, it had been merely a large drapery shop on the Left Bank, in St. Germaine. It was taken over by Aristide Boucicaut, and by the time he stopped expanding it in 1887 it occupied an entire city block. By 1914, it was the largest department store in the world, larger than Macy's in New York, Marshall Field in Chicago, and Selfridges in London.

When Zola set out the plan for his novel he saw the modern department store as a metaphor for modern life:

> *What I want to do in* The Ladies' Paradise *is write the poem of modern activity. Hence, a complete shift of philosophy. . . . Don't conclude with the stupidity and sadness of life. Instead, conclude with its continual labour, the power and the gaiety that comes from its productivity. In a word, go along with the century, express the century, which is a century of action and conquest, of effort in every direction.*

Like the film *You've Got Mail*, with its story of the small bookshop put out of business by a giant chain, *The Ladies' Paradise* depicts the destruction of the small drapers' shops in the surrounding streets. This was the agony and cruelty of capitalism, but for women, department store shopping represented a significant advance in their freedom and emancipation, for inside department stores, which were almost female-only zones of pleasure (and remain today largely so), women could spend a whole day, indeed have lived an entire social life, outside the house, without the need of a chaperone.

Zola describes the first modern forms of merchandising, the seduction and sucking in of the customer: advertising what was for sale inside; allowing free entry (no charge just to come in and look!), establishing for the very first time the principle of browsing, the notion of shopping as something you do for the pleasure of the activity rather than to acquire specific stuff; establishing fixed prices (no more haggling); allowing customers to return goods they aren't happy with; creating disorientation and apparent disorder of the shop floor, forcing the shopper to pass through many different departments to find what they were ostensibly looking for. All these were innovations of the department store. And above all, the department store established the idea of the shop as spectacle, of a visual theater, as Zola describes, "pleasures enticingly encased in their wrappings and sealed by the surrounding womb of warmth and light."

Plate-glass windows and electric light enabled the window display, and turned window-shopping along the grand boulevards into the activity of the flaneur. To be out on the streets, to be walking along and seeing objects of beauty and desire displayed along their pavements! To step inside the shops and to be enticed and flattered and offered the opportunity to drink a cup of tea and eat a cake, to have one's face massaged with unguents, to be attentively waited on by handsome young men in frock coats—was this not better than being at home with a Victorian paterfamilias, a Victorian-sized family, and a crew of maidservants to manage?

Shopping was attacked in the nineteenth century not because of consumerist materialism, but because it emancipated both the shopper and the salesgirls, releasing them from the physical drudgery of domestic service and placing them into close proximity with nice things: perfumes and scarves instead of coal scuttles and chamber pots. Inside the store was a world that husbands and fathers found themselves powerless to control or organize; a place with the first Japanese tearoom (Macy's in 1878), then a restaurant which took over a whole floor (Selfridges in 1902).

Men's public spaces were bars, restaurants, billiard rooms, and brothels. Women's public spaces were shops and beauty salons. With the restaurant and beauty salon inside the shop, women had a public arena of their own, one that men did not come into and weren't interested in coming into.

And although there were no brothels inside the department stores, women found in them a new sensual seduction. Such as at the glove counter, where Zola describes an erotic interaction:

> In the glove department a whole row of ladies was seated in front of the narrow counter covered with green velvet with nickel-plated corners; the smiling assistants were stacking up in front of them flat, bright pink boxes, which they were taking out of the counter itself, like the labelled drawers of a filing cabinet. Mignot, in particular, was leaning forward with his pretty baby face, rolling his Rs like a true Parisian, his voice full of tender inflections. He had already sold Madame Desforges a dozen pairs of kid gloves, Paradise gloves, the shop's speciality. She had then asked for three pairs of suede gloves. . . .
>
> Half lying on the counter, he was holding her hand, taking her fingers one by one and sliding the glove with a long, practised, and sustained caress; and he was looking at her as if he expected to see from her face that she was swooning with voluptuous joy. . . .
>
> "I'm not hurting you, madam?"

Shops, like cinemas, are dream factories. They sell glamour and illusions and unfulfillable desires. We see the goods, but most of them we can't have, yet it is usually enough to be among them, for a few hours. When I enter Selfridges on Oxford Street, I am hit in the face like a hammer with a throb of music. To walk along its vast ground floor, through cosmetics, jewelry, and handbags, is to take part in a great street party, one in which strangers offer to remake your face. If I jump into a cab and make my way to Harvey Nichols in Knightsbridge, I walk into a more quiet and discreet zone, where an edited selection of fashion is available to examine closely.

The point, for me, is to be in proximity to clothes. To see the things that are in the magazines. To gain some understanding of fabric, texture, and color. To hold a navy coat up against my chest to see if the shade of blue drains me or brings some warmth to the skin. To try on a Donna Karan jersey dress I have no intention of buying because I want to understand why people rave about the cut of her clothes and how she does draping.

To shop with no aim to buy is to immerse yourself, for a few hours, in fashion. We civilians don't go to the shows, we have no access to the ateliers. We will never own an Hermès Birkin, but we can look, feel, experience. This is an *actual* Balenciaga dress. You come close to the source, the origin of what fashion is, the mutable mysteries of time and pleasure, the whole crazy changing world of style with all its moods and excesses and sudden surprises. For shopping is not necessarily the point of going to the shops. It's a meditation, a frame of mind, a therapy, a balm for the troubled soul. Better people than myself might sit under the great dome of St. Paul's and contemplate God and infinity. Good luck to them. When I travel, I rarely take in the sights, especially if they involve staring at a transept, a nave, or some other bit of church architecture. Not to mention ruins.

If you want to understand the life of a foreign city, how people go about their day-to-day business, what they buy and what they look like, go to the supermarket. I rarely have the need to purchase a box of breakfast cereal or a loaf of bread while abroad, but watching others do it tells me more about a place than being led around in a queue behind a tour guide's umbrella.

⤳

I think of shopping methodology as the difference between hunting and gathering. To be *in the shops* has nothing to do with shopping, it's just going to take a look, and this is the true pleasure of what appears on the surface to be shopping but is more akin to spending an hour or so in the National Gallery, wandering from room to room and educating one's eye. And it is different for men and women.

A man walks purposefully into a shop and wants to find, as quickly as possible, where they keep the shirts (preferably on the ground floor, as close as possible to the door so he doesn't get lost). He sees shirts. He sees shirts in his size. Initially bewildered by the vexing choice on offer, dizzied and blinded by excess, for in the wild there is only one type of mobile food around at any given time, he slightly panics until, stabbing a finger, he says, "That one." The shirt is taken to the cash register; he hands over money. He expects the price of a shirt to be stable across ranges, across designers, across quality of fabric. A shirt is a shirt. How much can a shirt cost? The shirt is placed in a bag. The transaction has ceased. He leaves the shop hurriedly. Shopping is over.

Possibly he will return home with the shirt, his wife will take one look and then return it the following day for a shirt which she will spend forty minutes selecting.

Of course, this is a gross and sexist generalization. Many men I know take as much pleasure in shopping as women do (and there are women who hate to shop), but it is women who have finely honed the gathering instinct which appears the moment they enter a shop.

There are two ways of shopping. One is a mission expedition, the search for the scarf with a bit of red in it to go with the navy linen jacket. Or a dress for a party. Or a new winter coat. Or that most exasperating of searches, for shoes you can actually walk in. The second is, as I have outlined above, not actually shopping at all, but an exercise in pleasure and self-education, just to see what is in the shops.

The mission shop is a military exercise. Suppose one has as the aim the purchase of a winter coat, which, one has decided, will not be black but a color. The expedition involves a survey of the winter coats and their styles this season, the length, the arrangement of the buttons (double- or single-breasted), vent at the sides or at the back. So that's one whole shopping trip, just to look at coats in general and get an idea of what's going on with coats, and what colors are around this year. Then, having arrived at what color you're looking for—say a deep chocolate brown—you start to try on coats.

It is axiomatic that the coat which is the right chocolate brown and the right style and the right length and which fits like a glove will be by Armani and costs £1,500 (about $2,400). Everything now descends in increasingly depressing order from that utopian perfection which you cannot afford. It has established itself as the Platonic ideal of coats for which you will spend the rest of the week (or perhaps your life) searching.

You try on coats. E. M. Delafield's description of shopping in her satirical work of fiction, *The Diary of a Provincial Lady*, published in 1930, describes this experience:

> *Try on five dresses, but find judgment of their merits very difficult, as hair gets wilder and wilder, and nose more devoid of powder. Am also worried by extraordinary and tactless tendency of saleswoman to emphasise the fact that all the colours I like are very trying by daylight, but will be less so at night.*

Shopping to buy is hard on the feet and hard on the nerves. Whatever you want, they haven't got it in your size, or it's the wrong color, or it makes your hips look like two ships' prows, nosing out from the harbor. Sometimes one is doomed to disappointment. You don't find anything you like. You wind up with second best. You take it home and think, *What* have I just done?

But why should shopping for clothes be any different from the rest of life, with all its sorrows and its occasional joys? This *is* life, not a scene from a *Vogue* fashion shoot, with all its airbrushed, Photoshopped, sample-size perfections.

Ultimately you will find a chocolate brown coat. And in the years to come, photographed standing on a cold day in early February beneath the Eiffel Tower, or stepping onto the Venetian vaporetto, or just posed outside your new house, you will puzzle over the strangers in the background, the man raising his hand, the crying child, the unfamiliar color of a front door you opened and closed for fifteen years, and you will say: "I remember that coat. It took me a week to find it but it was perfect. I'll never have another as nice."

The other form of "shopping," *just going to have a look at what's in the shops*, which forms a major part of my recreational or work-avoiding in-store activity, usually does not result in a purchase, unless it is of the order of general household maintenance: a replacement mascara or two cosmetic products bought because if you do you will receive, absolutely free, for nothing, a makeup bag containing samples of other products, half of which you'll give to a friend's teenage daughter.

Looking, studying, thinking. Possibly trying on. Can I wear red? Possibly, but which shade of red? Picking up an armful of red tops, dresses, coats, jackets, and holding them up against you, or better still, taking them to the changing room, will give you a significant advantage when you next think that you're actually going to buy something. A new season brings new shapes; you can't know if they'll suit you until you actually try them on.

●

Lately, perhaps under the influence of advancing age and economic uncertainty, I have started to shop not like a teenager but like a grown-up. Instead of saying, "Ooh, look, I've got to have it," I am starting to buy like a person not so much with caution but advance thought.

In a recession there is the temptation to stop buying clothes, and at first this can be superficially soothing, for the soul can sicken on consumerism, shopping and spending. There is a mother lode of comfort in making your own soups at home instead of going out to a mediocre restaurant to pick over a lukewarm starter slapped on a table by a waiter who is adding up in his head how much he's going to make in tips. With fewer occasions to go out, who needs to dress up anyway? The simpler life of jeans and T-shirt can seem a radical new approach to living, the clothing equivalent of moving out of the city to the country.

You look, with satisfaction, at the deserted shops. You feel the puritan virtue of the nonspender flowing like ice water in your veins. You sell off your collection of It bags and then close down your eBay account. You realize you have not bought a copy of *Vogue* for months. You have no idea what they showed in Paris or London or Milan. You do not care. You have no idea why Keira Knightley is wearing a demure high-necked blouse with a bow. You no longer have a clue. You have fallen off the edge of fashion and will have to be rescued at some point down the line by a pair of bossy posh women who will force you to look in the mirror at a middle-aged frump.

The you I am writing of is not me but a creature of the imagination because in a recession the last thing I want to feel is depressed, and depressed I would feel if I was wearing dreary, cheap clothes, if I had abandoned, in a mood of austerity, the very notion of style. So shopping must happen less often, but with more thought, for in an economic downturn you cannot afford to buy cheap, disposable clothes. And so in triumph, my family's two mottos (*Only the rich can afford cheap shoes* and *There's only one thing worse than being skint [broke], and that's looking as if you're skint*) echo like animated foghorns down the ages. You see, my grandparents actually were poor, it was not a temporary condition. And so they understood shopping more deeply than their shallow privileged grandchildren.

So I have a plan: to go and buy the most expensive and most beautiful winter coat I can afford, not the cheapest. A major designer fling, so every time I put this coat on, I know that I have wrapped around me a hedge against inflation, and later ruin. I like the image of ruined old women, sitting in their last mink in a café, smoking a cigarette and drinking a small, appetite-suppressing cup of coffee. I buy my coat against that potential future. Even if the lipstick bleeds into the cracks, at least we're seen. In a recession you cannot allow life to turn beige.

And last of all, the shops are free. Inside them, those glittering cathedrals of beauty, as long as you're properly attired, you are welcome. You need to buy now the costumes you will need for the impoverished future.

No fashion is ever a success unless it is used as a form of seduction.

CHRISTIAN DIOR

SEXY

I HAD LUNCH with the designer Avsh Alom Gur, who was putting together his collection for Ossie Clark, Spring/Summer 09, a label which sadly no longer exists. Another victim of the recession. We went up to his studio and he showed me fabric samples, sketches, toiles, and one or two finished garments.

"I call them my imaginary friends," he said, speaking of the dresses that inhabit his head. Friends that do not take on flesh until the cloth is dyed the right color, the right thread has been sourced, the people in the workroom have made up a sample, and then he sees them for the first time.

"Why are clothes important?" I asked him.

"They make a woman feel sexy," he said at once.

Such a strange word; you know instantly what it means, but what does it *really* mean? To look sexy, to stimulate desire in others. To feel sexy, to be confident in the skin inside the clothes.

Until that lunchtime I hadn't even been thinking about clothes and sexiness, nor had I considered writing about it. Women who dress for themselves do not dress for men. For as a friend once remarked, men look at a woman and see a fuzzy pink outline. Of course I knew that what we wear expresses, announces, and even shouts through a foghorn messages about our sexuality, but that is because men do not notice what women wear unless they drag around a huge illuminated sign flashing the word *TITS*. And many do.

But so decisive was Av's response that I was forced to consider that feeling sexy and looking sexy are not quite the same thing. You could put on a tight bustier, a body-con skirt, and towering heels and still feel like you want to go back to bed and die. For while it is quite true that clothes transform us, can make us into a wholly different person against our apparent will, because clothes always have the capacity to be costume, *feeling* sexy is dependent on more than our fabric friends.

If I look out of the window onto a city street, I cannot help but be inundated with images of sexy. Sexy is perfume ads, sexy is fashion spreads, sexy is movie stars on the red carpet on the cover of a magazine, sexy is the sight of young women waiting at the velvet rope on a Friday night in their pulling dresses and pulling shoes. Sexy is an organized series of simple messages: short skirt, low-cut top, loads of makeup. Anyone can be seen to *do* sexy, even if they're anesthetized from the waist down.

Once, in Bangkok, in 1989, en route to Vietnam to write about what had happened to the bar girls of Saigon, those comfort stations of the war, I asked to be taken to an authentic sex club. The bar girls had melted away into the postwar country or escaped on dilapidated leaking boats to the Philippines and Hong Kong. There were rumored to be prostitutes there still, servicing visiting Soviet dignitaries and Vietnamese party officials, but not the lascivious displays of human flesh on sale to sex-starved Iowa farm boys in uniform.

The Bangkok hotel concierge told the taxi driver where to take us. We drove through the steamy city. On a stage I witnessed the ping-pong act, a listless just-pubescent teenager taking down her white cotton briefs and moistly projecting the white balls from her vagina. I had never seen anything so upsetting in my life, for these doomed children, who could not be expected to survive the AIDS epidemic into their midtwenties, were *acting* sexiness. They hadn't a clue. To the eyes of a grown woman, myself, the harmless gyrations of the hips and twiddling of little button nipples were heartbreakingly fake. They didn't look sexy because they didn't feel sexy. They were following a mime script, one written for them by a middle-aged man.

Watching from the audience, I thought that if I had a magic wand, I'd turn them all into kittens, chasing playfully around the squalid stage after a ball of wool.

Simon Doonan, creative director of Barneys and onetime celebrity judge on *America's Next Top Model*, the reality show in which small-town homecoming queens compete for a modeling contract, reduced a contestant to tears by advising her to "go down to the docks, see what all the hookers are wearing and avoid it."

The girls, he pointed out, were not deliberately dressing to *look* sexy, but to conform to a current teenage trend which he aptly labels "porno chic." When the crying girl accused Doonan of calling her "a ho on national television," he tried to explain that he was merely advising that if she dressed like a porn star, she might be taken for a porn star. The contestants stood about looking mystified. Doonan "felt bad for them. They [were] ill-equipped to survive in the big city because they simply [did] not understand the significance of any of their fashion choices." Their clothes, he tried to explain, to their baffled incomprehension, were a form of nonverbal communication, and that people made assumptions based on the messages those clothes were sending out. If they walked about wearing outfits closely modeled on Julia Roberts's car-crawling ensemble in *Pretty Woman* then it would be assumed that they charged by the hour. (And if they dressed like *shlumps*, that usefully onomatopoeic Yiddish word meaning "slobs," so would they be judged.)

Did the girls on the show *feel* sexy in their porno chic getups, or were they simply copying Britney?

"All over America," Doonan writes, "people are making kamikaze choices about what to wear. They are misrepresenting the goods. They are letting their clothes write checks that their personalities cannot cash."

Dressing sexy is by definition superficial. The goods are on display. Sex itself is anything but. When one considers depths and surfaces there is nothing that is so distant from our rational minds as sex. For sex is a torpedo under the intellect, sex has its own ideas and its own ambitions. Proust writes that while the mind is still lying in bed, turning over the pros and cons of taking a railway journey, the will has already gone down to the station and bought the tickets. We are rarely in doubt about physical attraction. Sex makes the self-important brain passively impotent (crying out in indignation, *How dare you! Don't you know who I am? I have an opinion!*)

Sex is right there, in the center of us, like a clap hammer inside a bell tower, beating out its one Big Idea, and you would think sex's monodimensional simplicity would make it easy enough to please. But I think of it, in marine symbolism, like the portrayal by Bill Nighy in *Pirates of the Caribbean* of Davy Jones, with a writhing beard of serpents concealing most of his face. For many and weirdly various are human sexual attachments, including one man who became erotically drawn to his car.

When we dress to *feel* sexy, as opposed to dressing to *look* sexy (or as well as), we're doing something so complicated I can't even begin to understand it, and perhaps only a psychoanalyst could. We are going with our instincts, whether it's the suburban transvestite stealthily trying on his wife's evening gown or the woman striding down the street in full leathers (to state the rather obvious).

෴

Agnès b. showed me a photograph of a model in a skirt that fell well below her knee. All along the front were big buttons. But two or three of the buttons at the hem were undone. This, she said, was sexy. Agnès herself was wearing a black trouser suit, a black and white harlequin shirt, black pointed-toe cowboy boots. Her hair, blond and tousled, unbrushed, looked as if she had just got out of bed after many hours of vigorous lovemaking and had thrown something on to run to the office. She was sixty-six.

It is not the dress that is sexy, it is the person in the dress. Whatever she wears, Victoria Beckham is not sexy. Whatever she wears, Scarlett Johansson always is. And so is Helen Mirren. These are ineluctable facts.

For here is the odd thing about clothes: that while Scarlett Johansson and Helen Mirren will look sexy in a sack, the rest of us find that what we wear is like a light switch. It turns on and brilliantly illuminates what lies beneath.

We choose our clothes for all kinds of reasons: for their practicality (old jeans for working outdoors, a warm sweater on a cold day, a thin T-shirt in the heat); because we are obliged to follow a dress code (a suit, shirt, and tie at a wedding, the new imperative of business casual, a uniform if you're a soldier or policewoman); because we're interested in fashion (and must wear this season's —— and not last season's ——); in the knowledge of how to disguise the flaws in our figure and highlight our advantages (no waist, good legs); because they are comfortable (an elastic waistband).

But then there are things like the color red. Crepe de chine. Old velvet. Satin. Leather biker jacket. High heels. The drape of fabric so that it slithers over your hips. The sudden revelation of a waist. Curvaciousness. The undone button.

Sexy is not the desire to have sex. Sexy is not what turns on the person looking at you. Sexy is a state of mind, of understanding that under all the drapery there is a body, and inside the body are instincts and desires. Sexy is a state of being. It's a way of knowing you're alive. It's the sensual relationship of skin to cloth. It's the awareness of the distance or closeness of the physical space between yourself and another. Most of us, unlike Johansson and Mirren, do not look or feel sexy all the time, but most of us manage to bridge the gulf between looking and feeling sexy quite a bit of the time.

What Avsh Alom Gur meant when he talked about clothes making a woman feel sexy was that clothes make us feel like a woman, womanly, not a mind operating inside the bony cave of our head (as I feel most of the morning, when I am writing) or a harassed mother whose femaleness is defined by the presence of ovaries and their awesome powers.

Many women when they reach middle age, or menopause, cease to feel that they are women, or women who are endorsed by male attention. Their clothes announce their resignation; they've resigned from being women. They're resigned to no longer being looked at, so what does it matter what they wear, or what they feel, or indeed if they have any feelings?

And yet when Germaine Greer published her book *The Change*, she told a studio audience of menopausal women on breakfast television that they should rejoice! For now they were liberated from the humiliating status of sex object, liberated into passionately announcing that with menopause, they no longer felt like having sex, and no longer needed to pretend to dress as if they were sexy.

And was greeted by a baying howl of jeers and derision, as women demanded to know in whose name she spoke. Only hers. For they *did* feel sexy.

Looking at Av's dresses and tops in his studio, I was struck by how very little flesh they bared, and yet the colors (the acid yellow, the shimmering blues) and the way he had draped the fabric, in some way I cannot begin to understand or explain, made me feel that he understood what it was to be a woman, as Dior had done: "No fashion is ever a success unless it is used as a form of seduction."

I now believe, as I used not to, that without some element of muted sexiness women don't feel entirely themselves. Paul Poiret described the art of the great couturier as that of the painter who "intends to make of your dress a portrait of yourself, and one that resembles you." We can forget for many a long year to be or feel or look sexy. We can rebel against sexy as Germaine Greer has done. We can give up, or be too depressed or too downtrodden, but if you put a woman in a sexy dress and show her her own reflection in a mirror, she will first weep and then laugh.

Because it is necessary, this desire to be sexy; it's the deep part of who we are. It's all the difference.

And that is all I have to say about sexy.

> Our clothes are too much a part of us for most of us ever to be entirely
> indifferent to their condition: it is as though the fabric were indeed a natural
> extension of the body, or even of the soul.
>
>   ҫ QUENTIN BELL

OUR FABRIC FRIENDS

RECENTLY I POINTED out to a friend who had taken up a new job in a new city that she seemed to be spending all her money on designer clothes. I didn't know where the money was coming from, but that was none of my business. For I knew that from an early age my friend had only bought the very best she could afford, being a student of art history with what I call a "decisive eye": the eye that understands exactly what it is looking at and can make informed aesthetic judgments. She could not stand to wear cheap clothes, a trait she inherited from her parents. Her mother, growing up in Israel in the fifties, during times of great austerity, would be taken once a year to the tailor's to have two outfits made. By the time her own children were born, and living in London, tailors had been replaced by designer labels.

Her daughter says that her insistence on only wearing the best is purely learned behavior, but I don't believe it. Abhorring ugliness, she was offended by the sight of the second- and third-rate. And she could see inadequate clothes with a great visual clarity.

I envy the decisive eye, which I don't myself have, being less visual than aural, more responsive to music than to pictures, but I do understand that your primary perceptive sense must be the eye if you are to be really well-dressed. You have to understand color and form and proportion. You have to know how to really *look*. And it is not enough to stand before the mirror and get a general impression of yourself in the garment; you must attend to detail.

Either you are born looking or you are inculcated with this skill. Entire societies have trained themselves to acquire an eye. Dior himself made the observation in his autobiography:

> *On the whole the American women—with the exception of those who dress in France—attach less importance to the small details of fit and to the finish of the dress, than to the general effect of the whole outfit.*

This was very much the experience I had when I went shopping with my friend for a handbag. Where I just went "Wow," and handed over my credit card, she took an hour to stand with it first this way, then that, thinking about it from every angle, indeed thinking thoughts about a bag which have never entered my own head. It was all in the detail, such details that I fail to notice until weeks, even months later, when I stand in the bedroom thinking, What the hell's the matter with this thing?

Her eye, her taste, her exacting aesthetic was why she could not bear to wear cheap clothes from the high street. With her first earnings she bought herself a Prada wallet. I once misunderstood or misremembered something she had told me and suggested she had one or two things from H&M. She responded with hurt shock. There was a pair of trousers from H&M, it was true, but they were Karl Lagerfeld's collection for H&M.

When her little girl was eighteen months old, and able to start wearing real clothes rather than those bags with legs and poppers decorated with clowns and bunny rabbits (I'm speaking generally, of course—she would *never* put her daughter in clowns and rabbits), I bought her an agnès b. dress in which cherries with their own individual shadows were dotted against a white background. It was A-line, which seemed to me the correct shape for the big-bummed diaper wearer. I purchased it knowing that the child's mother would be starting her daughter out on the path she had herself followed (and her own mother before her)—an insistence on the very best.

Still, my friend seemed to be spending an awful lot on clothes these past few months: a couple of Nicole Farhi dresses, a MaxMara, a Rick Owens. Every time I opened my e-mail inbox there seemed to be another link to net-a-porter.com, so I could see her latest acquisition. I was bothered by this not because I begrudged my friend her beautiful dresses, or because I thought she was a spendthrift, but because she had by now convinced me of the little-but-best rule which she seemed to be violating with her continuous purchases and I was worried that I had not really got the hang of the system. So I cautiously e-mailed her:

To my knowledge you have bought five designer dresses this year–2 NFs, 2 Rick Owens and the Matthew Williams. Are there others? because you told me you hardly ever buy clothes.

She replied:

And there's the stripy Vivienne Westwood I bought after watching Sex and the City. *I admit there is something weird going on. I think it's because I feel lonely here (without girlfriends) that I am filling my life and wardrobe with fabulous fabric friends.*

Was it funny or sad that she was making a friend out of a jacket or a pair of shoes? When I mentioned it to someone else, who had also made a life-changing move some years earlier, she understood at once what she meant. For she felt that the clothes she brought with her were her only constants: the clothes were what she could depend on when everything else was in a state of flux. They were familiar objects from the past, reliably transported into the present across time and space. And the new clothes she bought were her companions.

They sit inside the closet, the shapes of people. They have their personalities—the chirpy little floral skirt like the chattering girl you can't put down or shut up; the mean, brooding, dangerous leather dress which will lead you over to the other side of the tracks where the bad boys are; the dependable jeans that hold and hug you, like an older brother; the ephemeral flighty blouse, that ever hopeful romantic. The severe black dress without ornament like a woman who sits in a café smoking a red-stubbed cigarette and draining a cup of scalding espresso, reading a copy of *Liberation*.

"Old clothes are old friends," Coco Chanel once said.

This is the sort of sentiment you would expect from Chanel, but the eighteenth-century French philosopher Denis Diderot touchingly explored his feelings for an old dressing gown he had abandoned, a dressing gown which, in its decrepitude, had fulfilled the function of both pen wipe and duster:

> *It was made for me; I was made for it. It hugged all the contours of my body—but comfortably, without construction. In it, I was picturesque and handsome. The new one, tight and stiff, makes a mannequin of me. . . . Protected by my old dressing gown, I feared neither my servant's clumsiness nor my own, neither sparks from the fire nor leaking water. I was the absolute master of my old dressing gown; I've become the slave of the new one.*

In Edith Wharton's 1905 novel *The House of Mirth*, the tragic Lily Bart examines what remains of her wardrobe as she descends from New York high society into the social and economic abyss. From wearing beautiful frocks, she's reduced to learning a trade, millinery, at which she is not adept, and is, anyway, only a small remove from prostitution. It is a horrifying novel, of what might have happened to the various Miss Bennets of *Pride and Prejudice* had they slipped off the edge of Jane Austen's miniature ivory world:

She had a few handsome dresses left—survivals of her last phase of splen-
dour . . . and as she spread them out on the bed, the scenes in which they had
been worn rose vividly before her. An association lurked in every fold: each
fall of lace and gleam of embroidery was like a letter in the record of her past.
She was startled to find how the atmosphere of her old life enveloped her. . . .
She put back the dresses one by one, laying away with each some gleam of
light, some note of laughter, some stray waft from the rose shores of pleasure.

Like a letter.

Clothes as text, clothes as narration, clothes as a story. Clothes as
the story of our lives. And if you were to gather together all the clothes
you have ever owned in all your life, each baby shoe and winter coat
and wedding dress, you would have your autobiography. You could
wear, once more, your own life in all its stages, from whatever they
wrapped you in when you emerged from the dark red naked warmth of
the womb to your deathbed.

As if the textile itself has memory, formed as it is out of its intimate closeness with our bodies, a coat or a dress or a pair of trousers is a witness to the fact that once we went for a job interview, or
on a hot date. Or that we got married. The dress was there with us,
it's proof of who we once were. The clothes we wear, they comfort and
protect us; they allow us to be who we want to be. They tell others what
we want them to hear. We come to understand whether or not we can
depend on them. There is the loyal comrade which, whenever we put
it on, behaves just the same as it ever does; it reliably is the same from
wearing to wearing. "I'm here for you," it says. "Don't worry, we'll get
through this day together and I won't let you down." And there are
those fickle acquaintances that sparkled at a party a month ago and
now, released from the wardrobe, in a fit of pique insist on being
too tight (when nothing else you have is too tight), or weirdly having
changed color into a shade which doesn't suit you. Or taking on the
sudden appearance of that shopping catastrophe, the mistake.

Do our ways of looking at ourselves change, or does the actual dress itself change? I sometimes wonder if it's the latter. If they do not really have secret lives of their own, snuggled together on hangers or folded in drawers, gossiping about you behind your back and those loyal retainers speaking up in your defense. Or so I hope.

These ties of the heart have little to do with what the designer intended when, say, Karl Lagerfeld in his Paris atelier sat down to make a sketch. The designer is engaged in an epic lifelong struggle with space and time, to master a piece of cloth and form it into something new, because fashion is all about the new. That is its point. But the great designers leave on their garments, like a lingering scent, some part of themselves. Christian Dior tried to explain what he did when he designed a dress:

> Fashion has a life and laws of its own which are difficult for the ordinary intelligence to grasp. Personally, I know exactly what I must give to my designs: care, trouble and enthusiasm. They must be the reflection of my everyday existence, showing the same feelings, the same joys, the same tenderness.

Dior, a man capable of writing his own biography without reliance on a ghostwriter, was able to come close to the strange nonverbal realm of fashion in all its complexity. He was imprinting his own identity on his couture, perhaps not even imprinting, which implies to lay something down on a surface, but creating out of himself a kind of soul for the dress (if that does not sound too nutty). At least he understood that fashion involves not simply concept and abstract ideas but also human emotions. By observing what happened when he put a dress on a particular model (though Dior would not have used this word—the dress in those days was called the "model" and the girl who wore it the "model girl"), he was able to observe the transformative effect, not just of the dress on the girl, but of the girl on the dress:

Every woman invests a dress with her particular personality; thus a model worn by Marie looks quite different when Chantale wears it; one extinguishes but the other transfigures it. Having decided on the difference, I still have to analyse the reason for it.

Once his designs had left the collection, been made and sold, Dior would experience the odd sensation of running into them in the outside world.

For all this time I am meeting my dresses again. Like dear friends I meet them all the time at dinners and balls; a little later I meet them in the street—already getting further and further away from the original, because they are copies. Finally I discover them, major or minor travesties of my original conception, in the windows of the shops.

In the summer of 1971, I had perfect shoes. They were pink suede wedges with suede ties that did up around my ankles like Grecian sandals. They were the most beautiful shoes I have ever owned, and I was twenty and had no idea that in all the years to come I would forever be trying to find their replacement, as if they were a love tragically lost, or the Platonic ideal of shoes, or the shoes God had made specially for me. Whatever I was wearing, I only had to look down at my feet to know that they were encased in pink suede. I could and did walk for miles in them.

I had, that summer, little enough to attach me to the ground the shoes walked on. I had been sacked from my job in the press office of Oxfam for incompetence. I rarely showed up or I arrived late, in a stoned stupor. Collecting unemployment benefits, living in a rented room on an island in the middle of the Thames, an island large enough to contain just two houses, I drifted about all day trailing wafts of patchouli oil amid the stink of others' badly treated Afghan coats and joss sticks oozing an upward trickle of strong-smelling brown smoke. A summer of punting on the Cherwell. Riskily taking LSD on May Day, hearing what I believed to be the music of the spheres. Forecasting my future in the petals of daisy chains and the I Ching. Van Morrison, Pink Floyd, Sandy Denny. Laura Ashley dresses, dresses run up out of striped Indian bedspreads, crushed velvet jackets, jeans frayed at the hems and with a triangular insert of paisley cloth stitched into the flares, hennaed hair.

I wore the shoes every single day, until they fell apart and I dropped them in the kitchen garbage bin in an act of affirmative confidence in the future: that I was only twenty and that for the rest of my long life there would be other shoes—the next pair of shoes—but there was no next pair of shoes, none as good as those. Never again would I have a pair as beautiful and wearable. It must have been in part their pinkness but also the wedge and the thongs they were tied with which all combined to make them stand outside time, outside the era they came from. The point about those shoes is that I could wear them right now, today. So the past goes on tormenting you, the memory of brief intense friendships with shoes—yes, *exactly* like a lost love.

If I could dress myself now in anything I wanted, I would be wearing those shoes.

Or perhaps I am just trying to convince myself that I used to be twenty. You feel twenty inside your head, but then you look in the mirror and the reflection stares back at you, that dreaded stranger. If only I still had the shoes.

◌◌

Aged twenty-seven, I had a flat stomach, a narrow waist, and no tits. Many of my clothes that year were bought at a secondhand shop, what we now call "vintage." The name above the window was Joe's Old Clothes and it smelled of exactly that: old clothes, their sweat and dust and grime, and the sweat and whiskey of Joe himself, who was, I think, Ukrainian. The clothes were hunched together on rods, grim and crowded, like the passengers in steerage on their way to the New World, except for them the journey was not heading into the future but to oblivion.

The shop was on a main road leading into the center of Vancouver. From the west you could smell the port, the sea, the cargoes. It lay between Chinatown and Skid Row, where crippled alcoholics from the logging camps went to drink and in a few months die of cirrhosis of the liver and TB and later AIDS.

Despite the unpromising circumstances (you took a deep breath and held it in before you walked inside), some of the most beautiful clothes I have ever owned came from Joe's. He had curtained off a corner as a dressing room and fixed a mirror above it, from which, if he bent his head at the right angle, he could see the girls stripped down to their underwear. A few blocks away another shop sold horsemeat, which I believed he fried in a back room for his lunch. I don't know anything about him, whether he was married, how he got into this trade, what sort of a living it gave him, or how he acquired his stock. I suppose that something interesting had happened to him in the old country during the war, but you would not have wanted to ask. You were in and out as quick as you could, and his prices were very reasonable, considering what marvels that grimy Aladdin's cave contained.

Around two months ago, after an invasion of the clothes snatchers (moths) in my attic, I was forced to open an old suitcase that smelled of damp and mold, and inside it was a skirt I had bought at Joe's. It had once been a New Look dress of a particularly vivid turquoise satin with pale blue sprigs and a boned bodice which stood out from my chest, as empty as a Christian missionary's collection box in a mosque. A friend with dressmaking skills, which I, butterfingered, have always lacked, simply took the top off, threw it away, hemmed the waistband for me, and now I had a skirt. Because of my little waist, it sat on my hip bones, and sometimes, when I dieted, I could push it off with my thumbs even without unfastening the zipper.

When I took it out of the suitcase I could just about do up the zipper, with effort. I did not realize that I used to be thin.

That year, 1978, I was doing an MA. I earned a meager living as a graduate teaching assistant, leading seminars in English literature. The campus had once been crawling with student and faculty revolutionaries, and there were still any number of American draft dodgers, entering their thirties and still looking for trouble. One day the university support staff went on strike: the secretaries who typed out the course descriptions, the laughing women who doled out the slop in the student cafeterias, the silent men who swept up the cigarette butts in the lecture halls all marched out.

They set up a picket line on the approach road to the university, which was set on a small mountain onto which the clouds came down on winter days so you really felt yourself to be in a tower of ivory. It was an honor and principle not to cross the line. Solidarity with the workers! From early morning we flung ourselves in front of Mack trucks driven by squat teamsters smoking stogies, shouting up at the cab: "Don't be a scab!" In the afternoons we held frenetic organizing meetings; in the evenings we went to the pub, drank too much, smoked till we made ourselves sick, and then went home to practice various forms of horizontal trade union recruitment, leading to the occasional sign-up to the Trotskyist groupuscule of the day, headed by those rangy handsome Americans in their Levis, leather jackets, and boots. Marriages broke up. Women hooked up with other women. I went shopping.

I had no cash at all, we were all flat broke, but if there was a spare moment from the struggle I tried on clothes just for the hell of it. I went to Eaton's, one of the chain Catherine Hill had worked for, and worked my way through the suede jackets; it didn't matter what the price was—if you can't afford to buy anything you can try on whatever you like. Such as a black sweater, short in the waist, with ribbing on the shoulders and flecked with turquoise sparkling thread. The sweater cost $34, which at the time was, for me, a high-ticket item if I had been getting a paycheck, but I had nothing. So I got an application for a credit card, was approved, and bought it.

The sweater exactly matched the turquoise skirt, and I wore it all the time. You wake up in the morning and ask yourself what you should wear, and the seductive whisper of the same outfit you wore yesterday is in your ear: "Wear me." And you do because you know you look good, you look fantastic, but more significantly, you look like yourself and not an impostor.

I remember that summer. When it wasn't raining we went skinny-dipping on Wreck Beach, walking down a tortuous path to reach the sand where people lay around undressed and you could buy home-made piña coladas from an enterprising hippie with a bottomless thermos. When the sun went down, we gathered wood and built a fire and danced around it, lit up like imps and devils in the red glow from the flames. The draft dodgers talked about Vietnam and civil rights marches and the women goaded them about women's liberation. But you just had sex anyway, because it was there, lying around, waiting to be had. It wasn't a problem or an issue or something which needed to be discussed. You were naked more than you were dressed, absolutely unself-conscious, assured, with the piercing clarity of those who believe themselves to be absolute masters of the future.

Did the union win the strike? I have no recollection. Eventually, at the end of the summer, we returned to work.

I was teaching a class of undergraduates; I don't recollect what course. Romantic poets? Too clichéd but possibly true. There was a boy in my seminar, nineteen years old. He looked at me from under brown eyelashes and blushed. We went for coffee and then I invited him to see a film at the art house cinema and we returned to my apartment.

"I knew this was going to happen," he said as his tongue made some initial, exploratory licks.

"When did you know?"

"You turned to write on the blackboard, the first day, showing us the proper use of the apostrophe in *it's*, and when you reached up, that black sweater with the turquoise sparkles rose up over the waistband of your skirt and showed your midriff. It was so sexy."

"Where do you buy your clothes?" he asked me later. And I told him that the sweater came from a department store and the skirt from a junk shop.

I have never thrown away that sweater. It fits, just about, but I can't wear it in case I raise my arm and it exposes my midriff. It's still there, folded, among the Brora cashmere sweaters and the Gap T-shirts. But I take it out from time to time and look at it, just a piece of cheap acrylic and cotton knit, nothing special. I think, "That's who I really am, folded in that drawer, and the person in the mirror—she's the thief who came in the night and stole my face, my body."

The boy contacted me a few years ago. He was in his forties and life had not turned out for him as I would have expected.

Sometimes clothes are more than clothes, and throwing them away is too much like an amputation.

Recently I took the skirt to the thrift shop because it was too beautiful to keep locked up in the moldy darkness. It should have a third life, as someone else's skirt, passed clear over into the new century—I bet the woman who first bought it never foresaw that. It's the only one of its companions which emerged from the factory to survive so long. Someone had designed it, another woman had sewn it, a third had sold it, a fourth had worn it, then me. All long dead, I suppose, and Joe himself. I wanted it to go on, after twenty-five years shut up in the dark.

It's vintage, I tried to explain, but the two women at the counter looked at it as if it were a *schmatte*. You don't understand, I said, but they just smiled, coldly. I think they threw it in the recycling bin and I walked down the road feeling like a murderer. Which is cracked, because it's just a bit of cloth, but it still upset me, and I looked at the clothes that remained in my wardrobe and wondered what would eventually happen to them. They had been kinder to me than some people I know.

❦

I have in the wardrobe a heavy, black shearling coat. Twice on a December morning in Manhattan after an overnight snowfall, I slipped on an icy sidewalk and went down on my hip. So weighty was the coat that I only felt a small bump as I hit the ground. The coat was as good as a suit of armor protecting me from the enemy of the winter street. It's a wonderful coat to wear when I am feeling vulnerable, or when I need help beyond my own resources. It also makes me look rich, a rich middle-aged woman in a fur coat, which is not a style we are used to seeing these days. But I have earned the right to wear that coat; I worked my fingers to the bone in the service of words, the English language, tap-tap-tapping on the keyboard. I look in the mirror and see a middle-aged woman, and yes, damned right, she deserves a fur coat. Even if fur is out of fashion. She deserves a coat that will save her from breaking her hip.

I don't wear it as often as I used to—the winters do not seem to be as cold and it's a little big—but I have resisted every temptation to sell it on eBay. Like a dog, or a husband, or the teddy bear a child places at the foot of his bed to guard him, the coat is the reminder that when I feel its weight on my shoulders, I'm strong enough to bear its sumptuous load.

Though this morning what I want more than anything else in the world is a black patent leather stamped mock crock shearling flying jacket, of such an obvious vulgarity and fuck-you insolence that only a middle-aged woman (or older) could carry it off. With a violent slash of red lipstick on her ageing face.

Fashion always occupies the dividing-line between the past and the future, and consequently conveys a stronger feeling of the present, at least while it is at its height, than most other phenomena.

∽ GEORG SIMMEL

FASHION

ONE OF THE MOST perplexing aspects of fashion is its preoccupation with change, and hence with time. Its mutability is the point. Even those who take (or claim to take) no particular interest in clothes will, by accident or passivity, nonetheless go with the fashion flow. A man who wore a doublet and hose in the sixteenth century will not be wearing such an outfit in any of the following centuries unless he's on his way to a costume party. You would either have to take great care of what you already own so you rarely needed to buy new things or go looking for passé ones to be completely out of fashion, which takes more work than being in fashion.

We can date old photographs by what people wore, how they styled their hair, the contours within which the women drew their mouths. If we were to propel ourselves back to the twenties, we would notice at once that there were only three available shades of lipstick, and only one style of hat, the cloche. Only the elderly, those resistant to the new silhouette, would appear to have a waist.

How people are dressed is the most reliable indicator of differing periods in history. Not architecture—I live in a house built a hundred years ago. The whole street was thrown up at the turn of the last century. A variety of cars of various ages and models propel themselves across it. But the people walking along the street tell me that it is the spring of 2008, and a cold late spring, because young girls are still wearing the uniform of this winter: a short, colored, double-breasted pea coat worn over opaque tights and slouchy boots.

Fashion is all tied up with modernity, for fashion is always about what is now, of the moment. Even when it raids the past for influences, it updates, never simply copies. Ourselves in clothes are in the process of being and becoming. We dress for our lifelong journey *through* time, the transformation of the self, a recognition that we are in thrall to the ticking clock. Nothing more cruelly reveals the business of our ageing flesh than sticking to the same clothing, makeup, and hairstyles for the whole of our lives. And nothing reveals the passage of time more decisively than looking back at the clothes we were once able to wear, the size of them, the amount of flesh we self-confidently allowed them to reveal.

Clothes mark out periods in our lives. When I see old pictures it embarrasses me that often I don't know who the other people are, posed on a sunny day on a small rectangle of cardboard, everyone clearly enjoying themselves and happy in each other's company, or pretending to be. Who *is* that young man with whom I am exchanging flirtatious glances? What was so funny to make me throw my head back and laugh? Why does that unknown woman have her arm around my shoulder in a show of affection? And whose dining room table are we all sitting around and whose birthday are we celebrating, and who is that baby?

But I have never not remembered or recognized what I was wearing.

The ability always to recognize my clothing in old pictures is not so surprising. For the period of their lifetime as my clothes, one way or another I saw them every day, either wearing them or rifling through them on my way to finding whatever it was I was going to put on. The people in the pictures were often barely known, acquaintances. On them my life did not depend. There is nothing worse than getting halfway to work and realizing that you are wearing the *wrong thing*, the garment that you are not in the mood for or which expresses an aspect of yourself which is not the one you are trying to put into play that particular day. Or it's torn or dirty. Or just wrong for the occasion.

Where the clothes in the pictures subsequently went to is a mystery I don't like to think about. They vanished like the people in the photos. Indeed, clothes do have a habit of disappearing without a trace before they are worn out. I sometimes think they secretly leave the house under their own steam, late at night. A friend told me that as a child she had been forced to listen to a bedtime story, a cautionary tale about a little girl who did not look after her clothes, and feeling neglected and unloved, they ran away while she was asleep and went to live in the wardrobe of another, tidier child. You could give a child nightmares with this scenario.

⁊꧇

Much of our interest and absorption in clothes is to do with pleasure, a pleasure revived by Christian Dior after the war, and never since felt and seen with such intensity. That was Dior's gift, to make you fall in love with clothes. But the twentieth century is pinned by two names, Dior and Chanel, poles apart, rivals, the opposites of each other—one about lavish display, the other about severe simplicity. Each suited a totally different body shape. One emancipated women, the other imprisoned them again in corsetry. Yet we cannot have one without the other. And it is Chanel we must study to have an understanding of fashion and how it rides the crest of time.

The first thing to say about Chanel is that she invented modern dress.

I don't say that without Chanel we would all still be wearing ankle-length skirts and bustles, because the forces of history, of the twentieth century, and of modernism would inevitably have given us the silhouette we now take for granted. Someone else would have done it. But as it happens, it is because of the person called Coco Chanel that we do not walk around looking as if we were on our way to Queen Victoria's Diamond Jubilee, in vast skirts and huge hats.

Why? The hemline. There is no known period in the history of clothing after the Bronze Age and before the 1920s in which a woman showed her legs, let alone her knees, but you could put on today Chanel's little black dress from 1926 without turning heads. This is the puzzle and the paradox of her work as a designer: that she made clothes so radically new that no one had ever seen anything like them before, and at the same time their very newness seemed to stop time in its tracks. "A fashion that goes out of fashion overnight is a distraction, not a fashion," Chanel said.

Chanel was not the most imaginative designer of her era—that honor goes to Paul Poiret, who made some of the most beautiful and innovative clothes of the twentieth century. *He* is the forgotten genius who almost single-handedly liberated women from the Victorian corset, who created the world's first designer perfume, and who was the first couturier to create an entire lifestyle based on furniture and interior décor.

At the turn of the last century dresses were rigidly fitted to a woman's form: the bum jutted out at the back, the breast jutted forward. What women wore resembled not so much clothing as upholstery. In photographs of the period the women of the Edwardian era appear buried under their dresses, a small oval of face under dyed, frizzed, artificial bangs, peering out from the textile immolation of a high collar or pearl choker. No wonder the wealthy required maids to help them dress, to hook up bodices, lace corsets, button boots. Decoration lay heavily over decoration; a woman's true shape was unimaginable.

This was what Poiret altered beyond recognition. After working for Worth, the Dior of the nineteenth century, he set up his own house in 1903. Two years later he married Denise Boulet, a young provincial girl who was said to never have worn a corset or high collar. Her slim figure ("Like a lance in repose," one observer remarked) became the template for a Poiret garment. A fragment of film from 1911 shows her looking utterly different from the crowd she moves among—as well as being married to a designer, she was her own stylist.

With Denise as his muse, Poiret's dresses and coats fell from the shoulders and instead of being fitted to the body flowed along its natural lines. In inspiration, they were a throwback to the style of the Directoire, the period of the Empire line a hundred years earlier, but they were not pallid imitations—he canceled every existing rule of clothing to create the blueprint for modern dress. Culottes, harem pants, shift dresses, dresses cut along the lines of a chemise— his imagination stopped nowhere and prefigured almost every design innovation to come. But he did not foresee what was to replace him in the House of Chanel—the severe, the uniform, the pared-back, the minimalist, and above all the little black dress. For Poiret adored sumptuous fabrics and peacock colors; he described throwing into the "sheepcote" of insipid pastels "a few rough wolves; reds, greens, violets, royal blues that made all the rest sing aloud." Denise would step out to the shops wearing a wig of kingfisher blue and viridian-green stockings.

Almost everything Poiret touched was revolutionary. He seems to have invented the baby-doll nightdress, which would not return until the 1960s; he made dresses with asymmetrical shoulders, he introduced the hobble skirt, and even more startlingly, one of the most bizarre fads ever to be seen on the catwalk, the 1920s lampshade dress—a triangular tent with fringes hanging from the bottom, which, as *Vogue* wrote, every woman in the country bought.

Poiret designed for rich women. His sumptuous parties such as his legendary Thousand and Second Night ball were gatherings for everyone in the contemporary art world, for he was an early enthusiast for modern art. The three hundred guests were required to dress in oriental style or leave their own clothes behind and step into one of his own creations at the door. The painter Raoul Dufy designed fabrics for him.

Poiret's lavish tastes came to a grinding halt at the beginning of the First World War. He had to close down his house and go into the production of army uniforms. Discharged from military service in 1919, he reopened but discovered that the war and a generation of younger, enfranchised women had radically altered tastes. Fashion was moving into a period of mass production, which had never been Poiret's forte. The manufacturers were eager to clothe millions of ordinary women because that was where the money was.

The beginning of the twenties saw the arrival of clothes that were fit for the new roles that society had grudgingly offered women, which war had liberated them to play. This radical social change in women's lives and jobs profoundly affected fashion. Poiret was unable to adjust. He had always operated on a fine line between art and dress. Art inspired him, his clothes are breathtaking because of their incredible beauty. To wear a Poiret evening coat, no less than a Fortuny gown, is to be separate from the rest of humanity; it is a couture of vision and ideas. Yet by the midtwenties his frocks looked strangely dowdy, and it is a perpetual mystery how something that looked so right one minute can look so totally wrong the next. So wrong that you would cringe to leave the house in it.

Poiret's marriage broke up, the house went bankrupt in 1929, and after a brief and unsuccessful collaboration with Liberty in London he died in poverty in 1944 in occupied Paris. He was reduced to working in a bar and making his own suits out of tea towels.

(In 2005 a forgotten cache of original Poiret garments made for Denise were auctioned in Paris and twenty-eight of them were acquired by the Metropolitan Museum in New York. Volume and fluidity were Poiret's legacy to the future and that is exactly what we saw on the catwalks the season after the cache was discovered.)

So Coco Chanel did not arrive from nowhere; the groundwork had already been laid. But still, Chanel was the real revolutionary, the

Lenin and Trotsky of contemporary dress, the ruthless commissar, laying waste to the past, canceling it altogether, as if by some photographic technique she had managed physically to erase from the streets the waist and the ankle-length skirt. Middle-aged women had to go to Jeanne Lanvin for the figure-forgiving *robe de style,* which hid some of the body's deficiencies.

No one did more to lay down a style so enduring that it remains with us eighty years later. Chanel's work as a designer can't be separated from modernism: from Picasso, Stravinsky, James Joyce (and made more universal impact, on people who had no idea what modernism was, had never seen a painting or read a novel or heard a symphony). The underlying idea was the radical reinterpretation of reality, of altering its form in order to change its content. Cultural historian Elizabeth Wilson points out that early 1920s clothes "simply imitated [the] angular, two-dimensional style" of modernist painting with its emphasis on space, light, and color. But Chanel's "fashion nihilism" was the first to question, as art had done, fashion's own terms. As cubism or futurism were art for the machine age, so were Chanel's little black dresses.

Geniuses don't pay any attention to what other people think. They have their own, usually brand-new thoughts.

Chanel started life as an illegitimate child and grew up to become a shopgirl, and from a shopgirl, a mistress. French mistresses of the period are familiar to anyone who has read Proust. They lay in bed until noon, then went shopping. They lived to consume and be consumed, egging on their lovers to buy them jewels which would see them through to their derelict old age. Their milieu was luxury, and luxury goods, wallpapers, chairs, clothes, plumes. Chanel's biographer, Edmonde Charles-Roux, explains that once she became a kept woman, in with a horsy set, she started to have her clothes made by a local tailor whose only clients were huntsmen and stable lads. Charles-Roux thinks that "By dressing according to her own ideas, endeavouring in every respect to be the opposite of what those around her saw as luxury, Gabrielle [her real name] hoped to avoid the fate she dreaded most: being known as a kept woman. She already believed so strongly in the *costume* that she imagined all she had to do was not to wear it to avoid being cast in the *role*."

Chanel was still a provincial nobody when a new lover, the Englishman Boy Capel, moved her to Paris in 1908 and set her up with a little milliner's shop. Her first hats were relentlessly simple: "a wide waving brim with an almost invisible crown supporting nothing at all." No ostrich feathers or vertical plumes or cabbages of crumpled tulle or streamers. In July 1914, Chanel made her first outfit, using two fabrics which had barely left the locker room of sporting Englishmen and men of the turf: jersey and the kind of flannel used to make blazers. Machine-made jersey, which she discovered two years later, was intended for undergarments, long johns, vests. She made dresses from it.

Charles-Roux writes that Chanel was always ready to take the credit for Poiret's innovations, for the release from the corset and the shortening of the hemline, but it was, she concedes, Chanel who, in 1916, "made such decisive changes in fashion that she compelled it to change centuries: women had the right to be comfortable, to move about freely in their clothes; style became more important, to the detriment of adornment; and lastly 'poor' materials were suddenly ennobled, which automatically made possible the rapid growth of fashion within the reach of the majority."

The woman who dressed in Chanel, she writes, "bore no resemblance to anything, having—at least in their eyes—no memory and no tradition. She was an absolutely new woman, a woman whose dress was *without allusion*."

When she created the first little black dress in 1926 Chanel designed something of such radical simplicity that it was fashion's equivalent of the wheel or the fork. The black dress existed before Chanel turned her attention to it, but it was not little. It was mourning attire, and anyway, who could actually see it, buried under bows, pleats, lace trim, bustles, and leg-o'-mutton sleeves? What Chanel came up with was a dress that was minimalist, sophisticated, elegant. She advocated what she called "austere luxury"—the essence of chic. Her revolutionary approach to design meant that the black dress could be worn as daywear, cocktail wear, and evening wear.

The first little black dress, the Ford of dresses, was designed to be democratic; any woman could wear one whatever her social station. You could wear it to lunch at the Ritz and you could wear it to sit in the typing pool. The original design shows a long-sleeved, slim-hipped garment, gathered low at the waist and reaching to just below the knee. Its only adornments are two pleated V's dropping from the shoulders and rising from the hem, almost an exercise in cubism. Chanel would continue to develop this ubiquitous concept for the rest of her life, altering the fabrics, adding sequins or chiffon trains, but the under-lying simplicity remained. And this was hell for the first middle-aged women to put on the Chanel shape, for the whole newness of this very newest of looks in millennia was that it suited women who were new too, new in age—that is, very young, without hips or bosoms. When fashion became brand-new again in the sixties, it was the same thing. Clothes for the adolescent body.

⁓

I am not attempting to offer a theory of fashion or an investigation of the academic thinking on the subject. I have only a passing inter-est in it because what I really care about is what I myself wear, and not so much about what it all means. But when you lie on the sofa with a cup of coffee, vaguely looking out the window, wondering what you are going to put on tonight and why nothing you have in the wardrobe seems to be right (the age-old "I've got nothing to wear" lament), your thoughts inevitably turn to why it is that you cannot wear the fuchsia pink Paul Smith for Emma Hope embroidered jeweled velvet kitten-heeled mules that, when you bought them eight years ago, your hand trembling as you handed over your credit card, whispered seductively in your ear: "Investment dressing."

You can't wear them because kitten heels are out out out. Wrong wrong wrong.

But why should it be so? This really is a deep question and does require some understanding of the theoretical writing on what is called History of Costume.

The French critic Roland Barthes wrote a whole book on the "language" of clothes. Open it and you will find that "the more serious problem (because it is more specific) with regard to fundamental errors in all existing Histories of dress, is the methodological recklessness that confuses the internal and external criteria of differentiation."

Years ago, while a doctoral student in English literature, I used to read this kind of thing for pleasure, excited and exhilarated by the high levels of oxygen in the intellectual atmosphere. Now, not so much. Elizabeth Wilson, in her book *Adorned in Dreams: Fashion and Modernity* (1985), very usefully for me, did the hard intellectual spadework of analyzing why so many of these joyless theories of fashion don't hold up to scrutiny, especially when they are advanced by those with no personal interest in the subject and, what's more, are motivated by a fixed ideological framework, such as Marxism.

There is a desire, she writes, to explain fashion away and in reaction, for it repeatedly to have to justify itself. Intellectuals have been maddened by what they perceive as fashion's irrationality and labor to provide some functional reason for the most absurd of trends (like Poiret's lampshade dress). Or they claim that fashion is a capitalist plot, and that changes in styles of clothing are "foisted upon us, especially on women, in a conspiracy to persuade us to consume far more than we 'need' to."

The basis of this critique (and I hear it day after day from scornful men and some self-satisfied women) is that we have "certain unchanging and easily defined needs"—that having bought a pair of trousers you shouldn't need another pair until the first ones wear out, and there's no reason to buy anything other than an identical garment. And would do if consumer capitalism did not drive you mad by discontinuing the eternally useful and fit-for-purpose.

These arguments are based on the idea that we make logical decisions about what to wear. If we drift off this sensible course it is because we have succumbed to the narcotic of an oppressive society. And if only we could stop shopping, cease our endless search for unnecessary *stuff*, we could change the world!

But fashion is largely to do with pleasure, and pleasure is not rational, for we do not choose to eat, say, a chocolate éclair, with the aim of fulfilling our daily calorie quota. We fall victim to a cake because it is delicious. Interestingly the angry rages against unnecessary clothes are seldom replicated in moral campaigns against flambéed cherries or steak au poivre. No one pickets restaurants or rails against the conspicuous waste of unnecessary calories in a three-course meal, or the functional superfluity of cake. It is pointless fashion, not pointless cuisine, that gets the moralist's goat, and you would have to be pretty dim not to sniff the stench of misogyny that surrounds their outrage.

In a prelapsarian world, before Eve, temptress and first fashion victim, forced us to wear clothes, we got on without them. If it was cold, we cut the fur off our food and put that on. Or so the moralists have led us to believe. But Thomas Carlyle, in his philosophical satire *Sartor Resartus*, pointed out in 1831 that

> the first purpose of Clothes . . . was not warmth or decency, but ornament . . . for Decoration [the Savage] must have clothes. Nay, among wild people we find tattooing and painting even prior to Clothes. The first spiritual want of a barbarous man is Decoration, as indeed we still see among the barbarous classes in civilised countries.

The Old Testament holds many fascinating accounts of what Bronze Age peoples wore. During the period of wandering in the desert, while

Moses was up on Mount Sinai receiving the Ten Commandments, the children of Israel used their own earrings to revert to idolatry:

> And Aaron said unto them, Break off the golden earrings which are in the ears of your wives, of your sons, and of your daughters, and bring them unto me.
>
> And all the people break off the golden earrings which were in their ears and brought them unto Aaron.
>
> And he received them at their hand, and fashioned it with a graving tool, after he had made it a molten calf: and they said, These be thy gods, O Israel, which brought thee up out of the land of Egypt. (Exodus 32:2-4 AV)

There is, then, no golden age when people dressed entirely for function. Adornment has always been part of human nature. For as far as you can go, back into antiquity, the human race has done what it can to find objects and use them to make the body look better: more powerful, more attractive, drawing more attention to the erogenous zones.

Perhaps the earliest urges toward decoration had their origins in the relationship to the gods. Elizabeth Wilson argues that "when we look at fashion through anthropological spectacles we see that it is closely related to magic and ritual." Clothes, she suggests, put the individual into a special relationship with the spirits or the seasons. You do not wear your everyday clothes when you want to invoke a deity, especially when he or she is in the position to grant you a good harvest and save you and your tribe from death by starvation. Nor to be interviewed for a new job or to get married.

The atavistic urge to decorate the human body is a drive so immutable that no one has succeeded explaining it away by theories of capitalism. The question of why we enjoy dressing up is as profound as why the first man or woman made music out of a reed or drew pictures on the walls of a cave.

I'm grateful, too, to Wilson, for dealing peremptorily with the novelist Alison Lurie's critique of clothes as "largely unconscious aspects of individual and group psyche, as forms of usually unintentional non-verbal communication, a sign language." Lurie, Wilson writes, is "always the knowing observer, treating others to put-downs from some height of sartorial self knowledge and perfection." Wilson, in rejecting these explanations, comes to see fashion in all its perplexing human contradictions as about the way we both move with and through time, and how we attempt to defeat it.

Our bodies are changing cell by cell, molecule by molecule as we sit and breathe and I write and you read. We are in a constant state of transformation, first growth, then decay. Our bodies are the most mutable things we possess. Our minds and memories live inside them, prowling in the dark, humiliatingly dependent on the flesh-and-bone encasement.

Elizabeth Wilson cites German sociologist René König, who, she says, "sees fashion's perpetual mutability, its 'death wish,' as a manic defence against the human reality of the changing body. Against ageing and death. . . . And fashion not only protects us from reminders of decay; it is also a mirror held up to fix the shaky boundaries of the psychological self. It glazes the shifty identity, freezing it into the certainty of image."

Fashion is about the constant motion of time, and a defense against time. Only rarely do certain items of clothing, such as the trousers of blue denim, toughened with rivets, to be worn by laborers in the California gold rush, invented by German-Jewish immigrant Levi Strauss, attain a state of permanent fashion stability. There is never an era when jeans are the wrong thing to wear, though there are fluctuations in the width of the part that falls below the knees and the level of the waistline. Classic Levi 501s are indeed both modern and classic. It is possible to make a choice, as some men I know have done, to start wearing Levis or Lees or Wranglers in your teens, with a denim shirt and a leather jacket, and forty years later still be wearing the identical outfit, given replacements for wear and tear.

But most fashion isn't like that. James Laver, the fashion historian, anatomized the fluctuations of change:

The same costume will be

INDECENT . . . 10 years before its time

SHAMELESS . . . 5 years before its time

OUTRÉ (DARLING) . . . 1 year before its time

. . . SMART . . .

DOWDY . . . 1 year after its time

HIDEOUS . . . 10 years after its time

RIDICULOUS . . . 20 years after its time

AMUSING . . . 30 years after its time

QUAINT . . . 50 years after its time

CHARMING . . . 70 years after its time

ROMANTIC . . . 100 years after its time

BEAUTIFUL . . . 150 years after its time.

Are we dictated by fashion's whims, its short-term memory, its teeny attention span, its boredom, its love of the shock of the new? Or is fashion dictated by the human desire for change? There is a primal need for newness. Women get weary if forced to wear the same shabby dress.

The profound desire for something new perhaps is linked with the strong urge we have to be alive, just to be living. Unconsciously we understand that to live is to be in perpetual motion, and motion propels change. Fashion is always moving; its tendency to abandon abruptly a particular hemline, or color or style of jacket, or even a whole way of thinking about how women dress, getting rid of gloves and hats and pearls—fashion's maddening short-term memory takes you farther and farther away from the past. And if the past has not been good to you, you might thank fashion for making it look so firmly out-of-date, so old, so decisively not the present tense.

When we *cannot wear* a pair of kitten-heel mules because they are out of fashion, we are acknowledging that we can't live in the past. A few, a very tiny few, style eccentrics have always managed to break all the rules and wear what they want when they want, but the rest of us make those minor and major adjustments more or less unconsciously. Like great herds of bison thundering across the American plains we proceed onward, always moving on in packs to the next pastureland, or whatever it is that bison eat.

How do we know to adjust? Because of all the signals that surround us, in advertising, in films and TV, in what we see the celebrities wear on the red carpet, but far more significantly, what we see other people wearing on the street. We note not just what the most fashionable wear, but what the mass of the rest of humanity on the bus or at work wear.

Time past, time present, and time future are encapsulated in what we wear, our mutable identities constantly finding expression in a dress or a pair of shoes.

CATHERINE HILL:
DINNER WITH ARMANI

SHE WAS WITHOUT hesitation or fear. She was planning a boutique, a *European* boutique. Her first stock was from Umberto Ginocchetti, an Italian knitwear designer who had produced knits for Ungaro and Valentino, and was starting out under his own label. She bought five hundred items. He gave her some slacks to sell with them.

In Paris, near the Opera, she saw a little boutique with merchandise she liked and asked if they could let her have a few things. She bought cocktail dresses and some glamorous dinner coats with fox collars, the kind of thing that Marlene Dietrich would wear, and at $2,700 those were her most expensive pieces. But really what she was selling in those early years was what was just coming to the upper-class women of Toronto, a modern way of dressing; going out without the pearls and the little suit—the end of the Jackie Kennedy look.

The shop on Yorkville opened on December 7, 1972. Her daughter, Stefani, would come in after school to work, and she had an alterationist, a chain-smoking woman who could make a dress fit without actually knowing anything about fashion. So Catherine asked her to sit behind the desk, answer the phone if necessary, but otherwise not to speak to anyone. The first customer on that first day was an Italian woman who wanted a dress for her daughter's wedding. Catherine showed her the Parisian cocktail dresses. The woman said she would leave a deposit and take one away to show her daughter.

"I never owned a shop, what did I know? It's insanity to lend somebody a dress. At Eaton's we used to give out clothes but people always signed for them. But she came back and bought the dress. Then a man came in and he said, 'I want to buy something for my wife, it's my anniversary.' I showed him the evening coat, my most expensive piece, and he said, 'I'm buying it.' So my first day I had sales."

Catherine had insisted on having a yellow carpet. She had not thought about the street slush brought in on the feet of shoppers in a Toronto winter. She put up a discreet sign at the door asking customers to take their shoes off and provided the plastic slippers you get when you're having a pedicure. All over the city, at the high-class cocktail parties, the gossip was about Catherine Hill, that woman from Creeds who had opened a store with unusual sweaters from Italy, and who does she think she is? You can't go in without removing your shoes!

For the girl who had been in Auschwitz, who had left a loveless marriage to strike out on her own as a single parent with her daughter, and who had suffered the painful blow of rejection from Creeds, being in her shop, surrounded by the clothes she had bought from Europe, was itself a form of therapy. Clothes might not erase memories, of ugliness and brutality and horror, but at least they could be a kind of balm and comfort.

Some survivors of great trauma find a refuge in music or painting or literature or creating a garden or years of therapy. For Catherine it was enough to be among beautiful clothes. There, she says, "I achieve a serenity, nothing is jarring, my soul is full. Because there is something about beautiful things, it fills you inside. What you perceive with your eyes is just like the countryside or the lake; there is a melody that is nothing jarring about it."

The walls were papered in the then-fashionable cork, a chandelier hung from the ceiling, and she sat behind a desk a friend had designed for her. Just by being inside Chez Catherine every day, whose decoration she had overseen so that nothing she looked at was ever ugly, she moved far away from the cold, homeless refugee girl in her thin sandals who had made landfall in Nova Scotia, or the wife whose husband told her what she could and could not wear. Or the fashion director whose boss would not let her take those leaps of fashion instinct which are how fashion itself moves forward, by someone seeing or thinking something new.

But it was not enough to establish a shop and stock it with the designers she believed in. She had to be able to sell, to know her clientele. Not just to understand from the inside out what a woman wants, but to dismiss what she wants, the safe or unflattering option, and teach her how to dress. She learned the art of the great salesperson, the ability to help a woman find that dress which enhances her, which gives her, inside, the deep pleasure and self-confidence which we crave in new clothes. The decisive *yes*!

There was a certain tact which she had noticed in the saleswomen in Paris (they were exceptionally good at it at Dior) which allowed them to gently persuade a woman out of a garment that was wrong for her, but when Catherine, with her famous directness, saw that a customer had put something on which did not suit her, she spoke her mind: "You must take it off because it's not for you."

"I never waited for a woman to say 'I hate it.' I had this honesty that I had in my early childhood and I think I carried it right through to the business sector, and the customer felt that I had confidence, and they knew I cared, that I wouldn't sell them the wrong thing. Because I'm able to edit clothes in a showroom, that was my forte. You go in and see four hundred samples at Ungaro. You have to buy the line a certain way and I had disagreements with them because I wanted to edit it differently. I didn't want my shop to have exactly the same Armani pieces as everyone else. Joan Burstein at Browns in London bought a certain way, and someone in New York bought a certain way. Of course, there are certain signature pieces you had to have.

"So this strength I had in editing at the designer showroom I brought to the customer, instead of her floundering around. My store became very big, I had seven thousand square feet—they said it was like coming to a beautiful museum, so I didn't mind when they browsed. I think I loved the New York customer best, the ones who were born and brought up in New York and came to my Palm Beach shop which I opened later. I could always distinguish between Boston or Kentucky or Chicago, because the New Yorker has seen it all, they've traveled—they have a lot of department stores in New York, and they spend a lot of money."

When the British version of this book appeared, I did a reading at a literary festival and a woman in the audience raised her hand. She said she was a psychotherapist, and in the course of seeing many depressed patients, women who had little self-esteem, she sometimes thought that instead of the "talking cure" they might be better helped by going to see a good department store stylist who would bring some color into their lives and show them they were beautiful. There were those, she said, who could have done a lot better simply going to see Catherine Hill.

Catherine understood how women's self-confidence could be built up by the right clothes, and that a stylist was no less than an expert in teaching women to love themselves: "A woman comes in and says she's too fat. Suddenly she's diminishing her own worth. I remember I had this client, a Hungarian psychiatrist, and she adored clothes. She was going out with a younger guy and she used to lay out her clothes every night for what she was going to wear next day to the office. Even she was lost, and she had a good figure and everything. Because clothes don't have much to do with intellect. It's not how brilliant you are.

"In selling there is so much emotional giving. You go to a psychiatrist and the person lies on the couch and the psychiatrist takes notes. The involvement with dressing a person is that she is on your couch but you have to do all the work and talking because she's complaining about everything and you have to fix it right then and there. You have to take action, you have to do in one hour or twenty minutes the work that people go for two years to a shrink to get."

She also realized that the saleswoman (what they call in France the *vendeuse,* an important and valued aspect of the fashion business, far more than a mere shopgirl) is as much an actress as a therapist. "Selling is a constant performance, a theatrical performance, because you want the person to believe. There's a context, there's a play, there's a meeting. There's a beginning and then there is the final act and it's supposed to be a happy play. The only time it was difficult was when you have these beautiful things and the person is not the right size and you really can't help them. But alteration is a major importance, you have to have the best alterationist. Never have an expensive shop without it because that person has to know how to release and where and it's a moment of architecture, you're really molding that garment."

The saleswoman is a person who spends all her time observing others. She sees the strengths and flaws in a woman's body, she sees the personality they are trying to project, and if she knows her stock, and better still has chosen her stock for her customers, she can match the woman to the clothes, the clothes that express the identity. But above all, spending all day among women, the salesperson understands what it is to be a woman.

"I think the importance of what you're trying to write," Catherine reflected, "the importance of fashion, of what we put on, of how we try to present ourselves—nobody admits it. It is very important for women. They all want to look pretty, they all want to look secure, they all want to project something, and yet they say, 'Well, I don't care about what I wear,' and they're sloppy. I think they're denying something which is essential to a woman. It has something to do not just with femininity but desirability and sex and being appealing. You don't have to be vulgar, you don't have to be half naked, it's about the way you dress. And when men say they don't notice, I don't believe it."

After a few years, Catherine moved to a new store in Hazelton Lanes, a mall of high-end fashion stores with apartments above it, where she lives today. With a greatly expanded space, she began to buy seriously in Italy, particularly from three designers she championed at the beginning of their careers: Armani, Versace, and Ferre. A new development in retail, before the young designers opened their own stores, was for them to have small, stand-alone boutiques inside department stores or high-end fashion shops like Chez Catherine.

Initially there were problems selling the Italian designers. She had been buying Prada bags but when the clothing line came along, she found that they were not cut for the average North American woman. "The sizes did not correspond, a size eight was not a standard North American size eight. They were cut for the Italian figure and the Italian woman's figure is totally different, and different from the French woman, totally."

Valentino, Versace, Ferre, Krizia, and Armani all had boutiques in Chez Catherine and exclusive deals with her. It was terrifying and exhilarating, the sums of money involved. When Giorgio Armani opened his boutique in Chez Catherine she invited him to come to Toronto for the opening and he did.

"We had a wonderful luncheon in one of the empty apartments, right where we're sitting. We invited twenty-seven people, all the press, and he did not speak a word of English, so he got up and spoke and I had to get up and interpret everything because he always said, 'What do I need to learn English for?' I'm not sure until this day that he speaks English. So I had a very warm feeling for Armani because he's not only a beautiful person but his personality is genuine. Growing with them, they were like my children, I discovered them, they became famous. I found it very natural working with these designers. I always felt we were equals, and I think that the designers did not give me the feeling that I don't belong there.

"They knew that I was European and they respected the fact that I spoke the language. I always had the feeling with the designers that we were one family. When Ferre came to Palm Beach we went out disco-ing together, we had lunch and dinner together. He was the designer for Dior for several years and that's how I got the Dior label because as soon as he became the designer I automatically got Christian Dior.

"When he opened his boutique in Chez Catherine, I was having breakfast with him. I said, 'I am very nervous, I don't know what to do about the window when we open the boutique.' He said, 'I'm going to do something for you. We're going to get two or three hundred pink

peonies, then you're going to put the peonies on the floor in all the
Ferre windows. Don't put too much clothes, just a few here and there.'
He sketched it for me, he designed it over breakfast with the brioche.

"So there was a certain intimacy, when I was buying, when I was
in the showroom; the designers didn't seem foreign to me. I think
when I was at the shows I was in awe of the pomp and the elegance
and the people, because that is a fantastic experience, especially the
couture shows—that excitement when the lights go on and the clothes
come out. You see the effort and the talent which is so electrifying for
those twenty or thirty minutes that the shows lasted. I was transported
with them to this fairyland. The average buyer doesn't go to the couture shows but they all gave me tickets because I knew that what they
showed in the couture show really went down to the next season, so I
already knew what's going to happen six months or a year from now.
That was a very exciting period in my life, the shows.

"Sometimes you've seen a show and you knew that you're going to
have a harder time buying because of the period the designer was in—
they always wanted to bring something new in, and it's like skating
on dangerous terrain. You ask for different fabric, you had to be creative, your selection had to be very carefully done. Some seasons were
harder than others and some seasons were fantastic."

At this time, in the 1980s, Catherine had a lover in New York and
he persuaded her to open a store in Palm Beach, Florida. It was a
shrewd move, for many wealthy Canadians moved south for the winter, so besides attracting the American buying public she already had
a customer base.

"It was really the height of my career. I was acknowledged by my
peers in America, which was really what augmented my prestige.
The season starts at Thanksgiving and it finishes at Easter, so I was
able to close down my shop in the summer because there was a lot of
work: I had to fly back and forth, but by that time I had tremendous
staff there, I had twenty people working for me. It was a very exciting
period, between 1980 and 1990. Donald Trump offered me any space

I wanted in the Trump Tower, and now I wish I would have done a New York store, because I like the way the American woman makes a decision, I like the tempo. I would go to Jamaica and Nassau at Christmastime, and I met American children, and even at seven or eight years old they had to be faster thinking and make more decisions than the Canadian children. Anyone who is born in New York City, by the time she is forty, like the women in *Sex and the City*, has something about their thinking and decision making which is swifter."

The 1980s and the 1990s were Catherine's era, in fashion. The designers who emerged then are the ones she still reveres, and wears, today.

But there was always the occasional thought, as she considered the long journey she had made from Auschwitz to the front row at the couture shows, as to whether she really belonged there.

"We always went to congratulate the designers—myself, the president of Bergdorf's, Neiman Marcus. I usually made an effort to stand in line and congratulate them because I felt they worked so hard for the collections and they needed such reassurance. One time, as I was walking out after congratulating Valentino, I saw Linda Evangelista and she was wearing something with a stripe and I thought about the camp. Because of that striped thing she was wearing, I thought about Auschwitz.

"The glamour and the richness, the opulence which was such a contrast to my past—then there was suddenly a starkness, the world didn't seem real to me then. I was thinking about the values of the society, of the women who, most of them, knew nothing about wars. They had been born to wealth, they had experienced none of those things. Maybe they experienced sicknesses, but it's a totally different world. How lucky and fortunate they were that they were born in the right time and the right place and they never had to experience anything so horrendous as some of the European Jewish people did. The amazing thing is that I don't think any of my designers knew."

Catherine had her shop for thirty years. She sees that her life is marked by abrupt alterations in her circumstances, external events forcing a sudden change.

In September 2001, North American retail had been in a slump for several months, but the attacks on New York and Washington curtailed the desire to shop; fashion did not really begin to recover until a year later.

"That morning, when they called me from the store and they told me, 'Put on the television, there's something happening,' it was just like the world was going to fall apart. That day and after, nobody came into the mall. I had a tremendous anxiety and compassion for the people in New York but I felt that we're going to experience something bad again. It just brought back the Holocaust to me. It was horrendous, just like a war broke out in North America, and the people really stopped buying clothes. This I know because the retail scene was everywhere a disaster. Everything started to slide, something happened to my spirit. I had no choice but to close the store, especially as my lease was not renewed. I closed at the end of 2002. It was very traumatic for me.

"I think that closing my shop, it was like losing my home. It was a very similar experience to the war. I was free, I wasn't put in a prison, but I felt that everything was sliding from under me, I was drowning, I could not stop it. I had to close it because I couldn't find destiny, it was the same abrupt thing again. It was sad, very sad.

"People will say, 'Well, you could have made different choices, you could have handled it differently.' But you are shooting for the stars, shooting for the moon, and something happens. I feel very sad when I see the city, and I hear people saying to me, 'There will never be a store like yours.' There's no such thing, it's nonexistent. People appreciate me better now, they know the difference; it's really a pity that it could not remain the way it was, the exclusivity and the designers."

The long career in fashion was over, but what lay ahead was an attempt to understand the deep past, to make history comprehensible to herself and others. She had felt reborn when she reached Rome in 1946 and saw the lavishly filled shops, the abundance of food, the clothes and the reemergence of style, and she was indeed reborn when she made that long-ago landfall in Canada: reborn as Catherine Hill.

When she closed her stores, she wanted to reinvent herself, and that is when she decided to write her memoirs. In her retirement, she forced herself back in time, to fateful decisions that allowed her to survive. She thought and remembered.

When it had been duly impressed upon her that she was a young lady . . .
she suddenly developed a lively taste for dress. . . . [H]er judgement in this
matter was by no means infallible; it was liable to confusions and embar-
rassments. Her great indulgence of it was really the desire of a rather inar-
ticulate nature to manifest itself; she sought to be eloquent in her garments,
and to make up for her diffidence of speech by a fine frankness of costume.

— Henry James

MAKING A SELF:
THE CREATION OF I

In *Vogue*, I read an account of how author Elizabeth Kendall arrived at
Radcliffe from the Midwest in 1965 wearing an outfit she describes
as "a wrap-around skirt and a shirt." Quickly she realized she was
dressed all wrong, behaving all wrong, actually breathing all wrong.
By the end of the academic year she was enunciating her speech in a
bored wispy way, ascending the steps of the library in sling-backs, and
tucking her tweed skirt into an elasticated girdle, a garment which was
considered essential in the 1950s and early 1960s.

Wearing a girdle was a sign that you were an adult, whether your
flesh needed tamping down or not. It was armor and constraint. It
was womanhood, not girlhood. It drew your attention to your eating
and childbearing places, and kept sexual urges squeezed in check.
I remember this because very briefly, in my early teens, I wore one

myself, at my mother's suggestion. A girdle came soon after the first training bra.

At the beginning of her second year Elizabeth Kendall met a girl from California. She was wearing a sky blue coat and a straw boater hat when, Kendall writes, coats were supposed to be gray, black, or brown; in other words, utilitarian colors (but that is possibly because, marooned in Missouri, she had not seen what Givenchy, Balenciaga, and Dior had been up to in Paris throughout the 1950s, let alone Schiaparelli before the war). To Kendall, the whole outfit resembled a costume, and she was startled and impressed. But it was what lay underneath the sky blue coat that so entranced her: a tent-shaped dress made out of stiff canvas, "imprinted with huge red strawberries on a field of yellow." Kendall writes of this encounter:

> There are moments in one's life when a vast structure of assumptions shifts, opens, tumbles. [She] wasn't trying to look like an adornment to a Harvard man. She was a young woman whose every move proclaimed originality. And it wasn't just a pose. . . . The most potent of [her] traits, to a dazzled me, was the boldness that had led to that dress. Actually, she had several such dresses, all with different patterns. "You don't know about Marimekko?" she said.

Marimekko is a small Finnish fabric and clothing design company established in 1951 which had been featured in a 1965 issue of *Vogue* the year before this encounter. There was a pop art quality to the print they had chosen, black chevrons against a yellow ground on a simple shift minidress, and on the opposite page, a girl in a black and white bikini bottom with cutouts at the hips, a midriff-baring tank top, and flat boots in matching fabric. Elizabeth Kendall found their shop and a rack of dresses: "Each one," she writes, "was saying something like 'Rejoice!' in a language of huge fruits, psychedelic stripes, flower explosions."

When academics write about the language of clothes and describe the various messages that are encrypted in the garments, they seldom include in that vast vocabulary the word *rejoice*. Clothing as a social system is supposed to emit various significant social and cultural signals but not these piercing feelings of joy that new clothes can bring to the wearer. In general I prefer to those academic studies the modest maxim of the children's writer, Noel Streatfeild, who pointed out with simple but devastating precision, "There is no doubt a new dress is a great help in all circumstances." In other words, ask not what the clothes do in the world, ask instead what the clothes do for you.

Kendall stopped buying books in order to save for a Marimekko dress and after a few months went back to get one. It was covered with plum-colored sea urchins against a sea of rust-colored cotton, and its trapeze shape set her body free from the restrictive cage of the girdle. Looking back at those years at college, she writes, she sees herself always in motion, on a bicycle or running, in the Marimekko dress. She wore it to sessions with her thesis adviser, and this led to a dissertation on the then out-of-fashion novelist Edith Wharton, and writing about women writers, Kendall felt emboldened to become a writer herself.

Back home in St. Louis, she gave her mother her Marimekko dress for the simple reason that another girl in her dorm had given her *her* cast-off Marimekko, and it seemed that these dresses were made to be passed on, like a book which has changed you and you hope will change others. Her mother had recently broken out of the restrictive confines of 1950s American wifedom and got herself involved in the civil rights movement. A few months later, en route to a family vacation, passing through a storm, Elizabeth replaced her as driver. A truck passed them on the highway and drowned the windshield of the car with rainwater. Elizabeth braked, ran into a low bridge, passed out, and her mother, in the passenger seat, broke her neck and was killed.

In her late mother's wardrobe the Marimekko dress stood out against the sober costumes of the period, and her daughter took it back: "From then on," she writes, "I would wear it for both of us."

❧

At eighteen, most of us are frightened of individuality, particularly when we're a long way from home, among strangers and dying to fit in. There is, Kendall observed, a uniform, and she lacked both the self-confidence and strong sense of self which would allow her, like the girl in the sky blue coat, to ignore what everyone else thinks and wears. Teenagers *always* wear the same thing. Until a couple of years ago all teenage girls, whatever size and shape, wore low-rise jeans and short muffin tops, below which wobbled a roll of goose-pimpled puppy fat. Next they bought smock tops and skinny jeans into which legs like tree trunks were unconvincingly stuffed. They don't want to stand out, they don't want to be individuals. They, like Elizabeth forty years earlier, want to look the same as everyone else. From the basis of this conformity, most of us start to branch out.

We wear what everyone else wears, but that in turn is constantly undermined by changes which take place in society. In the 1950s, that "everyone" was in twinsets and pearls; a decade later, it was mini-skirts. The radicalized 1960s was a decade whose true and enduring revolution was the sexual one. Clothes were part of the physical liberation of the body, the undoing of what Dior had made twenty years earlier. Chic, elegance, style, femininity were no longer the measure of how you dressed. You dressed to feel free inside, and feeling free, perhaps you could actually make yourself (and others) free. You cannot take part in a demonstration in stilettos.

The freedom of sixties clothes, the liberating formlessness of the dress, the low-heeled, round-toed shoes, the dying away of the perm and shampoo and set (ruining my father's business) allowed women to be different kinds of women. It's impossible to imagine the women's movement dressed in the New Look.

Those who write about the language of clothes present it as an external conversation which exists only "out there" in the world. But clothes are always talking to us, and we are always answering back. Virginia Woolf, a feminist who never forgot about the importance of clothes, expressed this experience: "There is much to support the view that it is clothes that wear us and not we them; we may make them take the mould of arm or breast, but they would mould our hearts, our brains, our tongues to their liking."

This was the condition of my own immigrant grandparents who fled conscription in the Russian army at the turn of the last century to arrive, safely, on the shores of England. On arrival, my clever, resourceful grandmother, much brighter than her dreamy husband, who was always happiest with a glass of whiskey and a prayer book, looked carefully around at her new country, and observed that she and her family had no obvious position in the rigid doctrine of the class system. Which was an advantage, as no one could keep you down, tell you that you ought to know your place. And if you did not know your place, how could anyone know who, and what, you were?

For a gentleman wore a hat, a workingman a cap. Hundreds of tiny details about clothes sent out coded messages about the identity of the wearer. A lady had no need to wear an apron in the house; a maidservant seldom wore anything else. A working-class girl had boots on her feet; her mistress kid slippers. My grandfather, heavily bearded, looked at once like a foreigner, so he shaved the beard back to a mustache.

Simply by observing the dress codes of a class to which they did not belong, my grandparents realized that they could make their way in the world and dressed defiantly above their station.

They would come up with a number of family mottoes which would see them and their children in good stead in their attempts to integrate themselves into English society, find ways to earn a living, and steer clear of the authorities of whom they were very fearful, lest they do or say the wrong thing and be deported. Grandpa never learned more than a few broken sentences of English, but he did manage to express the following profound thought, which as I have said, is our family motto: "There's only one thing worse than being skint, and that's looking as if you're skint."

My grandparents had an innate understanding of the importance of clothes. Without a puritan bone in their bodies, with absolutely no longing whatsoever for the simple life, they instinctively realized that they would be judged on how they dressed, and the better impression they made as they moved upward in society, the better things would go for them. The six children of these two old people understood that clothes maketh the new immigrant. They spent a fortune on clothes. The men bought their suits at Austin Reed and the women demanded mink coats and diamond rings from their husbands.

Uncle Louis, my father's eldest brother, the most immaculate dresser in the family, took this a step farther, for he acquired a particular piece of almost existential wisdom. He insisted that whenever he bought a new hat his initials, LG, be blocked in gold letters on the sweatband. No one could see them, but with that hat on his head, with the important knowledge that the letters were there, leaching inside his own skull, he walked forth with greater confidence and swagger.

And, of course, when he took his hat off, to enter a house or to doff it to a lady, anyone could catch a glimpse of that LG and would know that there stood before them if not a gent, certainly a man who held himself in such esteem that his own name was written in short form in gold inside his homburg. And holding himself in good standing, others naturally took him at face value. For a while he made an excellent income in the sale of chamois leather which one used to clean windows and for other menial tasks.

Hence I grew up in a family home which knew a great deal about clothes while never being either at the forefront of fashion or in the clothing business. You gave a lot of thought to what you put on before you left the house. You used clothes as a weapon, as armor, as a means of gaining respect in the eyes of a frequently hostile world. If your clothes were out-of-date, then you would be judged accordingly: as someone who didn't have the common sense to know where hemlines

were supposed to fall this season. And if you had no idea about hemlines, what else might you not know? How naïve could you be about,
say, business? Was it possible to put one over on these rubes?

These were the commonsense values of my family when it came to
clothes.

As my grandparents found out, their clothing not only sent messages to the new country that they were themselves new arrivals, out of
place and out of time, but by changing the clothes (which changed the
message) they also changed themselves. Clothing was not just a disguise, though it could be; it also allowed the process of assimilation, in
which they became Englishmen and -women, to take hold. The chief
separation between my maternal grandmother and her daughter was
that the older woman, in ritual religious observance, shaved her head
and wore a wig, and my mother didn't. In fact my mother not only
went to the hairdresser's, she got a job as a receptionist and married
the boss. Not wearing a wig made her feel English on the inside, even
though English was not, in fact, her first language.

The belief that if you wear the clothes of what you wish to become
(or avoid the dress of what you don't want to be taken for), this idea
of putting on a costume to become the self you want to be, found its
truest expression in *vogueing* in the 1990s. Gay black men competed
with each other to walk down the runway dressed up as businessmen,
models, beauty queens, suburban housewives in the belief that simply
by showing that they could look the part, the part would inevitably be
offered them, however implausible they seemed. These were heart-
breaking ambitions. HIV-positive men from the ghetto, transvestites
who wanted the white picket fence and the husband, and knew exactly
how to dress the part. But it was a stretch too far. And yet they intuited that in the world they were shut out from forms did matter; they
had the courage of their convictions. Convictions, however, are never
quite enough.

The clothes you put on do not instantly make you the character you
want to be. Clothes are a lifelong journey into acquiring an identity,

an identity deliberately formulated, but also made by accident. You try on a tweed jacket and understand that it has connected with the part of yourself you scarcely knew about, which would like to go for a walk along a country road, with dogs. Or you put on a hat and discover in yourself a capacity to be quite lah-di-dah. And indeed all cross-dressing is a means by which we can give expression to those secret selves which lie concealed beneath our obvious appearance; who people believe us to be, but in our heart of hearts we aren't. Or not completely.

I developed my own identity through clothes, beginning with the velvet smock dresses which my mother bought me. If it was true that my mother had been a young woman during the war, had worn those short skirts, her hair in a roll, the clumsy platform shoes—then the war was precisely what she wanted to forget about as soon as it was over, having lost first a brother, then a fiancé on the battlefield. Let alone the nightly terrors of the air raids—she really wanted to forget about them.

The 1950s and all it involved could not come quick enough for her. The corsetry, the lipstick, the conical brassieres, the jewels, the alligator handbags, the seamed stockings carefully straightened before you left the house: all this hard work of being a woman—its preparation, its painful underpinnings, its cleverly maintained illusions—was precisely what she craved. She wanted to be standing next to my father in his evening clothes, a little sequined clutch in her hand.

And I sort of understood as a child that being a woman was about dressing up, that these were costumes, and indeed an outfit would be called a "costume." A dress was a frock or a gown. A suit was an ensemble. Clothes were not what you wore to be comfortable: they were how you built your femininity. Before her kidney-shaped dressing table with its triple mirrors, its drawers stuffed with her nylons, the central one with her palette of Revlon blue eye shadow, her gold tubes of Max Factor lipsticks, and her small bottle of Elizabeth Arden Blue Grass scent, my mother became a person who had an existence out in the world, not just inside the house. She made me realize that her inner identity was not fixed. That she could be something or, more worry-ingly, someone apart from a mother. My mother, in other words, had not just a life but an identity independent of me, and to that I was not at all sure, resentfully and with some anxiety, she was entitled.

I reached my teens at a seminal point, when couture was dying and being replaced by boutique, by Mary Quant, who had wept when, at my own age then, she had realized that she was about to be trussed up, choked, caged by clothing. At the very moment that I got to the point when I was ready for a scaled-down version of the "Bar" suit, there no longer was any "Bar" suit; instead clothes were designed exactly for my own still straight-up-and-down body. Those little tunic mini-dresses, those clumpy, round-toed shoes.

There is a devastating photograph, taken in the 1920s, of a wealthy middle-aged woman in one of Jeanne Lanvin's flapper dressers, creased around the middle from where she had been sitting down. What horror, too, for the women who, aged twenty in 1947, found themselves with hips and waists and bosoms at forty in 1967. To have to endure the boyification of the female form. But for me, aged thir-teen, it was just fine.

The defining moment in the life of a young girl is the moment when she is able to choose her own clothes. There are, of course, many other defining periods: first menstruation, first kiss, loss of virgin-ity, acquiring of contraception, passing your exams, leaving home, getting a job—yes, these are all monumental stages, but they are just stages. Milestones. Markers.

When you start to dress yourself, you are beginning a lifelong jour-ney into your own future, the subtle, everyday construction of who you are through what you wear. Of course, you come in at a particular moment in the fashion cycle, and where you come in will define what happens for the rest of that life. I started with miniskirts and trapeze-shaped dresses and American Tan tights. I thought the New Look was the exact opposite of its name—it was dated, old-fashioned, or in my mother's rather marvelous word, *antwak* (antiquated). As the film at the V&A would show, corsets were too hard to wear, corsetry was a relic of a prefeminist past—for old ladies, as Bardot had observed of couture itself. But at bottom, the New Look looked *all wrong*. Its oldness was too new. Because the worst thing you could do at sixteen was to dress anything at all like your mother.

Fashion was moving very fast; it was succumbing to extraordinary influences. Courreges, looking up at the sky and imagining men in space suits, put us in little white moon boots, and we came out the other end a few years later in *Bonnie and Clyde* maxiskirts and Biba feather boas. Because of the film *Tom Jones,* I wore my hair tied back in a low velvet bow. Because of Vidal Sassoon, my long hair was cropped into a five-point cut. Because of the Beatles and Maharishi Mahesh Yogi, I made a skirt out of a tie-dyed Indian bedspread and fragranced myself with a weird, stinking oil from India called patchouli. A decade later, because of punk, I bought a leather jacket covered in zippers.

All of these outfits were conditioned by both conformity and experimentation. It was agonizing to be out of fashion. As soon as a new style appeared you had to wear it, because you were, like fashion itself, in a continual state of flux. Fashion was a uniform, a code, which gave you safety in numbers; by fitting in with the crowd, the crowd you had selected, you were able to suppress your own insecurities. But every time you changed your clothes, you discovered another new self.

Epictetus, who lived between circa AD 55 and AD 135, advised: "Know, first, who you are; and then adorn yourself accordingly." But as we have seen, it is the clothes that allow us to find out who we are. Trying on, for example, a tweed skirt and pearls, I understood almost at once, looking in the mirror, that I wasn't that and this wasn't me (and still isn't).

But seeing a friend, returned from the hosiery department of Liberty department store in London with a pair of Mary Quant opaque purple tights, something I had *never* seen (only read about in D. H. Lawrence's novel *Women in Love,* in which the "bad" sister, Gudrun, wears colored stockings), I had a feeling that purple tights might be just up my alley. When I eventually got my own pair—and that was some hard work, requiring trips to London—I would go on wearing them, and their many replacements in many colors, for the whole of the 1970s. Colored tights came to define me, and certainly not because I had good legs to show them off, but because I felt that they set me apart from the sort of bland person who would wear flesh or beige-colored ones. They had a bohemian element and I wore them with clothes that we now call vintage, and then were just called secondhand.

They were already getting harder and harder to come by, these thirties tea gowns and cut-on-the-bias dresses, and the square-shouldered slim-hipped short outfits that had been thrown away in disgust by the previous generation when the New Look came in.

A place called Paddy's Market in Liverpool sold old clothes, and if you were lucky you could find the remnants of a rich old dead woman's wardrobe, but usually not, usually just old clothes. So I would get the train to London and go to the weekend market on Portobello Road or the tiny shops at Kensington Antique Market, where you still could, for a few quid, buy a crepe de chine evening gown. This was my style: the colored tights, the vintage dresses, the hennaed hair. This style was the summation of the identity I had been trying to reach through the various experiments which took place all the way through my teens. It was not entirely individual; many of my friends at university dressed just like it, with or without the tights (which might have been just a me thing). It was the style of university-educated girls with an interest in fashion, not much money, and a strong dislike for the trends of the 1970s—the tank tops, the huge collars, the browns and the oranges.

In the middle of the decade, I left Britain and went to live in Canada, where no one had ever seen anyone who had dressed like me before. I stood out like a sore thumb. What was wrong with jeans and a simple T-shirt? I was asked. I had no jeans and no T-shirts. I felt dehistoricized, a person without a past. They regarded me as an English eccentric, slightly nuts, but I had merely evolved a style out of the material available.

The midcentury novelist Ivy Compton-Burnett remarked irrefutably, "Appearances are not held to be a clue to the truth. But we seem to have no other."

Policemen, firefighters, judges, ambassadors, dictators, bishops, and admirals all have outfits to denote their jobs and their status. Take the horsehair wig off the British barrister, and all you have is a bald man with his mouth open. Take the army uniform off Saddam Hussein and what's left is an old man with a beard, in a hole.

A uniform is an easy way to announce to someone who you are, and an easy way to bury your own true self, as anyone who has worked at McDonald's can tell you. The magazine of the British Union of Fascists advertised to its readers in 1934 the transformation of their inner selves simply by putting on a black shirt, the costume of English Nazis:

> If you should join us, we will promise you this: when you have put on the Black Shirt, you will become a Knight of Fascism, of a political and spiritual Order. You will be born anew. The Black Shirt is the emblem of a new faith that has come to our land.

All thugs discover their inner courage in a uniform, knowing that it inspires respect and, more often, fear.

Grappling with this construction of the self through clothes, and the desire to express myself, I gradually realized, or returned to, what I'd known in my teens, that identities can be fixed or they can be ephemeral, an identity for a day or an identity which you keep in the wardrobe and bring out for various occasions. Or, as my grandparents intuited, they can be false identities.

When I open the doors of my cramped wardrobe with its jammed rods, the clear plastic bags containing cashmere sweaters, sheltered against the predatory attention of moths, the handbags in their own cotton bags, the folded jeans, the rows of colors (black, purples, greens, browns, navy, white), the coats, the dresses, the jackets, the tops, I see a frozen frame. Me, spring 2008. This is the size I am. This is what I own.

There are nostalgic items I do not wear but do not want to throw away, and there are things that don't fit, and things that don't suit me, and things that were always a mistake, and things I mean to wear but don't, and the workhorses of my collection such as this Vanessa Bruno dress and that Anya Hindmarch cream handbag.

Out of the items in the wardrobe I will select the items that will make up the self I plan to be that day.

But in the wardrobe there are also ghosts, absences, gaps, and memories. The clothes that I have owned have been an intimate and significant portion of my life. I have been another person when I wore them.

The idea that we find our identities and then express them through clothes in a series of fixed messages is to simplify a complicated process. It is not just that our identities change (when we start work, when we have children, when the children leave home) but that we ourselves are passing through time, and through fashion itself. And that what we wore at twenty-five can't be worn at fifty for a variety of reasons: because we look like fools, or because we have a new struggle, with our changing bodies.

The most fascinating and engrossing struggle a woman can have is how she is going to dress when she is old. And by "old," I mean eighty. When the old lady has such a low value in society, is so prone to stereotype, that the counteraction to those stereotypes by clothes is itself a kind of revolution.

I'll come to that.

From time to time I have come across people who *apparently* do not care for clothes, and wish they did not have to be bothered with them, apart from the primitive functions of covering themselves up.

I have met high-minded puritans in holed and stained jumpers, ill-fitting jeans, and Cornish pasty shoes standing on street corners hectoring us with the aperçus of their cast-iron moral and political certainties. All culture not in service to the higher cause of social progress is a form of false consciousness artfully designed to bamboozle the masses.

Or there are those who inhabit libraries warmed by the belief that an interest in one's appearance is a distraction from higher thought. The mind inhabits the body solely for the protection of its soft tissue. Caring about what you look like is for half-wits.

There are countless thoughts and aphorisms expounding this view: "Poets, artists, and men of genius in general, are seldom coxcombs, but often slovens; for they find something out of themselves better worth studying than their own persons" (William Hazlitt). And "Any affectation whatsoever in dress implies, in my view, a flaw in the understanding" (Philip Dormer Stanhope, 4th Earl of Chesterfield). And, I am sorry to say, from the novelist who never once stooped to describe what Elizabeth Bennet or any of her sisters wore to the ball: "Dress is at all times a frivolous distinction, and excessive solicitude about it often destroys its own aim" (Jane Austen).

I have some sympathy with women of the nineteenth century who saw the imprisonment of fashionable dress not only as an impediment to their freedom, but as a means of infantilizing their sex. To escape this catch-22, feminism, the movement which in my view was the most successful, necessary, and enduring revolution of the nineteenth and twentieth centuries, inevitably took a harsh view of women's preoccupation with clothes. Sarah Moore Grimké, the American suffragette and abolitionist, expressed the difficulties of women's advancement:

. . . [O]ne of the chief obstacles in the way of woman's elevation to the same platform of human rights, and moral dignity, and intellectual improvement, with her brother, on which God placed her . . . is her love of dress.

And a century later, the American feminist and novelist Erica Jong summed up the dilution of women's experience:

Isn't that the problem? That women have been swindled for centuries into substituting adornment for love, fashion (as it were) for passion?

The nineteenth-century campaign for Rational Dress, the initially eccentric wearing of divided knickers by the pioneer Amelia Bloomer, set itself in opposition to the voluntary immolation of women in garments and footwear and underclothes which were everyday instruments of torture. Victorian underclothes leave me aghast. Apparently upper-class women were unable to eat at those lavish dinner parties because their internal organs were so squeezed by tight lacing that it hurt to swallow. They ate in secret, in their bedrooms.

Madwomen can think remarkable things, and the idea of a woman wearing trousers, or swinging her legs over both sides of a horse instead of perching perilously on the edge of the saddle, her feet fatally dangling, was one of those concepts that I imagine to be born from unadulterated rage. The dehumanization of women through encasing them in body armor and icing it with lace frills can only be overcome by harridans and viragos and harpies—who moved on to even greater transgressions by dressing more or less identically to men, with trousers, shirts, ties, and monocles.

(And I cannot help but notice that while women can largely get away with wearing clothes only a degree or too away from male attire—jeans and T-shirts, differing only in the cut to accommodate the shape—men cannot wear women's clothes without being transvestites. I wonder why. And why do large heterosexual blokes get a frisson from donning silk panties? Is it because women's clothes are so far from rationality? You rarely find a transsexual trying on a pair of tailored Armani trousers and a matching jacket.)

But though I admire the campaigners who got us out of corsets, and while for a year or two in the 1970s I myself owned a pair of dungarees (they were in fashion at the time, what do you want from me?), the prejudiced belief that feminists are not interested in clothes is one of those urban myths born out of ignorance and malice.

Feminists, quite rightly, addressed one half of the equation: that if women were regarded as silly creatures who cared only about their appearance, by abandoning the dress codes which sent out that message they would correct the problem. In reply came the repressive response: women who don't pay attention to clothes are ugly.

Is it possible to defeat this conundrum? One can persist in saying that it is possible to be intelligent and dress well. But, of course, dressing well requires hard work, and for many male observers the work expended on the exercise is demonstrable proof of female inadequacy.

The solution to this aspect of misogyny is for men themselves to start getting interested in clothes and seeing how much effort it takes, and I'm glad to say that the payoff of consumer capitalism is that a younger generation of men have done exactly that.

◦◦

I live in London, which, if not the most stylish city in the world, is the place where you will find the most interestingly dressed people. For pure, unadulterated fashion pleasure you would go to Italy, where both men and women would not dream of leaving the house without a close inspection of themselves in front of the mirror and where the secret to their outstanding appearance is apparently down to the hours spent every day ironing. One of the drawbacks of the ATM is there is no longer a need to go into Italian banks and observe the

handsome men in beautifully pressed suits as they cash your trav-
eler's checks.

But London makes up for what it lacks in the natural unattractive-
ness of the English with its strong sense of urban life. In London you
know you are living in a city, and a city where you still shop on the
street, not at the mall, where you do not just step from your car to your
destination, where you move about on public transport, walk about on
genuine streets, and you are always being looked at.

Sitting on the tube, what stands out for me are the country mice,
the visitors to London who haven't a clue what to wear and who dress
for the occasion as if they were hiking in the Pennines or reconnoiter-
ing the Grand Canyon. Our city's permanent residents from Ghana,
Dubai, Bombay know how to dress. They understand the significance
of city attire, of how you exist in a megalopolis like London. As the
seasons turn you are imprinted with the image of the next big thing.
Everyone knows how to carry off a version of it. Everyone is trying.
Except the standouts, who aren't. Who haven't the faintest idea. They
think they can come to London and dress as if they were lounging
around the house at home but it doesn't work like that, not in a city.

I know that the world is full of the unself-consciously badly
dressed; no-nonsense types, doers, who make the world turn around
and put their efforts into something more significant than the fit of
their jeans. It is possible to invent Microsoft and Intel and *The Simp-
sons* while wearing truly dreadful clothing, not to mention campaign-
ing for a free Tibet.

But I have an instinctive tendency to recoil from such individuals.
I can see I am being looked over, with that "Who does she think she
is?" scornful stare, a tribute to their no-nonsense, forthright, non-
fancy-schmancy directness. In great swathes of America, dressing up
is the sartorial equivalent of the old class taunt "Who does she think
she is?"

Taking pride in being badly dressed, not caring how you look,
dressing to "feel comfortable"—these defiant fingers-up to civiliza-

tion are usually a pose. As Miuccia Prada noted, "I've become impatient when people claim they don't care about clothes. They still dress every morning, and if they are going to reject fashion, they still need clothes to show it."

∽

People tell me that they are no good at shopping. There are many, many things I, too, don't like doing and am very bad at, such as assembling flat-packed furniture, which, as Jackie Mason once pointed out with piercing accuracy, is something which people like me tend to do with the butter knife so once the item is made up we can still see the crumbs in the grooves of the screws. Being no good at shopping, panicky once you get inside the door, feeling overwhelmed by all the choice, is, I believe, a common disorder, like agoraphobia or fear of flying, and like them, limits life's possibilities. But there's always the Internet.

Then there are those (perhaps the majority) who take a utilitarian approach to what they wear, for whom clothing is about following a set of basic social rules so you can free your mind to think about something else. They have no philosophy about clothes. At a wedding they'll wear a suit. At a barbecue, jeans. At the beach, shorts. They appear to wear, broadly speaking, what is in fashion simply because that's what there is to buy in the shops. In the 1970s the bottoms of a man's jeans would have been flared, thirty years later they will not be. You'd have to either take great care of the clothes you already own so you rarely need to buy new ones or go looking for them to be completely out of fashion, which takes more work than being in fashion.

Those who take no particular interest in clothes will, by accident or passivity, go with the fashion flow. Appearing never to update their wardrobe, they nonetheless alter their dress over the decades, changes not necessarily observable to the naked eye because of the glacierlike slowness of their movement. We cannot watch a person ageing, but come back twenty years later and you will see the difference. Photographs taken over time will show subtle fashion alterations.

Others (and here I am mainly speaking about women) feel so miserable about their bodies that they make their purchases solely on the basis of what covers them up. They seek out garments, often in black and beige (the noncolors), or tracksuits, and send out a small whispered message. "Don't look at me." Or "It's what's inside that counts."

Then, of course, there are those who appear to take no interest in their clothing but who just have awful taste, with no idea whatsoever how to put an outfit together with some reference to fit and proportion and the color palette. They do care about what they wear but haven't a clue what they're doing. As Andy Warhol observed: "When I see people dressed in hideous clothes that look all wrong on them, I try to imagine the moment when they were buying them and thought, 'This is great. I like it. I'll take it.' "

I have very rarely met anyone who dressed badly because they could not afford any nice clothes.

To dress badly as a revolt against oppression, or as a political posture, has nothing to do with not being interested in how you look. Such individuals are constantly striking a sartorial pose. They are making big cartoony statements with what they wear.

In the past few years in London I have become used to seeing women on the streets who are making the biggest statement of all, the women who appear not to be wearing what I understand to be clothes at all but are dressed in the niqab, the all-encompassing garment which covers not just the body, but also most of the face.

Both the niqab and the hijab, the scarf, have been subject to legal and political interference, in Britain and in France, perhaps the first time in history when the state has intervened because a woman is too covered up.

The curious issue about Islamic dress is that it sends out a message which is usually a direct contradiction to what is going on under the swathings. If you see a woman covered up, you may assume she regards clothes as the work of the devil. Nothing could be further from the truth, as I observed in 1996 at a wedding in Iran where the female guests, sequestered from their husbands and other males, were released from their chadors and decked out in twinkly turquoises and pinks. There was little or no influence of Jil Sander or the other mini-malists.

At Selfridges, I have seen a dark cloud of women in niqab toting Chanel handbags disappear into the changing rooms with Gucci cock-tail dresses and Balenciaga blouses. I have faux-casually followed them in, ostensibly to try on something myself, but really to glimpse what they look like under the all-encompassing medieval black sheets, and have been startled to see a modern woman standing in front of the mirror, looking as if she should be drinking cocktails at the Savoy.

Islam does not suppress women's love of clothes, it displaces it, so it only exists within closely defined limitations, where it presses tightly against the walls of its restraints.

The teenage daughter of assimilated Muslim parents who chooses to wear the hijab as a statement of religion and culture is no more antifashion than the African-American men and women who in the sixties made a similar point by abandoning the scalp-burning hair-straightening chemicals and letting their hair grow out into Afros. "Look at me," those giant hairdos said. "Look at me." An assertion of self in a society in which they had literally a few generations ago been enslaved.

Were I a young Muslim woman in post-9/11 and post-7/7 Britain, I, too, would be considering how to use my clothes to make a point.

The only person I have ever come across who genuinely appeared to have no interest at all in how she appeared to others was a woman whose jacket hung loose off her shoulders as a result of weeks of not eating properly or sleeping. Her son had been killed. He was just twenty. She picked ineffectually at the encrusted food which stained her lapel, which she had only just noticed. But the next time I saw her she was in a black pantsuit, in public, speaking about her loss.

Washing your clothes, choosing them carefully are the first steps back to having a place in the world, and perhaps the ritual clothing of mourning (black in one culture, white another) is there for a purpose, to help us not have to decide what to wear.

When we return to life, when we look once again in the mirror, we understand without thinking about it consciously that to dress well, or at least appropriately, is to be in the world, and the world judges us on our external dimensions. You think you cannot go on; you find you have no alternative but to do so. You have to live. Caring about what you wear is one small but not entirely insignificant dimension of existence.

Mirrors should think longer before they reflect.

〜∘ Jean Cocteau

THE CLOAK
OF INVISIBILITY

A WOMAN IS standing at the reception desk at a hotel while the desk clerk is checking her in. A man goes up and tells the desk clerk he'd like to check out. She says, "I will be with you in a minute, when I have finished checking in this lady." The man turns in the general direction that she has indicated; he registers a chair, a plant, a picture, a door leading to the business center, an empty trolley waiting for the bellman to fill it with luggage, but he cannot make out a human form.

"I'm here," the woman indicates helpfully. Startled at the sound of a voice, his eyes try to focus on a faint outline near the desk. It is a sort of person, a visitation from another world, the world of unseen women over the age of fifty.

I have watched the eyes of men sweep a room and find that apart from the girl crossing her legs, over there, it is empty. After a certain age, women are invisible. Without a sexual stimulus, many men cannot process in the visual/conceptual portion of their brains that a woman is present.

And therefore, how we dress when we reach this age is more important than how we dress at twenty or how we dress on our wedding day if we want to have a presence in the world. If we don't want to be famished ghosts at the feast of life.

⟨∽⟩

My mother's generation was subject to stringent rules regarding what a woman could or could not do at a certain age. She must reach eighteen before she could wear her hair up. After thirty it was no longer permissible to have long hair at all. A lady wore gloves. She always wore stockings. She never left the house without putting her face on. At fifty, if she was rich, the reaching of middle age would reward her, in compensation for the loss of her youth and the privileges that went alongside it, with a mink coat and diamonds.

I have in my own wardrobe my mother's black Persian broadtail coat with its detachable white mink collar, its velvet-lined pockets, and her initials embroidered on the silk lining, which was scattered with rosebuds in tribute to her name, Rose. It was purchased from an East End furrier in 1959; the pelts are the skins of unborn lambs. Ewe. I have never worn it, on account of having its modern-day equivalent, my Nicole Farhi shearling, but I feel that I am entitled to it, both as an inheritance and by virtue of my age. I have grown into it.

In insurance terms it is worth a great deal of money—it would cost perhaps £10,000 (about $16,000) to make a replacement coat of that quality today—but a similar coat, for sale on eBay for £39.99 (about $65) attracted not a single bid. This is because fashion has turned against fur, but also because we no longer reward a middle-aged woman with a mink but with Botox or a face-lift. Still, I don't think my mother, standing at a hotel reception desk in her Persian broadtail in 1959, age forty-one, would have been a sight unseen. Her generation, at least the women who liked clothes and fashion, deplored sloppiness of any kind. They worked ladylike chic for all it was worth. You would not see my parents on their annual visit to London dressed in windbreakers, shorts, and huge shoes with Velcro tabs, heaving small backpacks, like a party of mature anthropologists on a field trip.

For the condition of many women who have reached fifty is to abandon the whole damned business, to turn conclusively to the color that will ensure that they are as transparent as a sheet of glass: beige, which in my opinion only suits Italian women with very glossy black hair and olive or lightly tanned skin, and looks worst of all on the washed-out English rose complexion, matched with salt-and-pepper hair cruelly cut too short, with short bangs and two little points above the ears.

I would not have expected this resignation from my generation, the one which, as I have said, believed in the 1960s that middle age was a lifestyle choice on the part of our parents, and that we were the first set of people born to be young and stay young forever. Others, true to their generation, have adopted a different response: to defy the whole ageing business by proudly announcing to everyone they meet that they can still fit into the same clothes they wore twenty-five years ago and that they and their daughter are always swapping jeans and tops.

If you had asked me in 1970 when did middle age start, I would have suggested thirty-five, and this would have been more or less accurate. Yet Mick Jagger, who has turned sixty-six, has not yet exhibited any signs of entering middle age. I suppose this is because middle age is as much as anything else a state of mind, and some people arrive for their first day at kindergarten with wise little faces and are immediately appointed classroom monitor and by thirty will be turning you down for a line of credit.

Nonetheless, I am prepared to concede that I am in middle age. I just wish it was called something different. The concession arrives from what one can and cannot wear. It's not a matter of seeking permission from others, or feeling you should be obeying the rules, but rather if you care about what you wear, you want to try to look your best, and in certain garments you do not. And it is the absence of rules that throws us into our contemporary uncertainty, which would have been unknown to my mother, who knew exactly what she could and could not wear, having discovered the neat little collarless jersey Chanel–look-alike suits in the early 1960s and worn them ever since.

She never in her life owned a pair of jeans. Trousers, polyester garments with elastic waists were what you wore around the house to do the vacuuming. As soon as she got home her best clothes were immediately taken upstairs and rehung on the hangers in protective covering. They were bought to last a long time, and did. In the early 1990s I persuaded her to buy a pair of leggings. Looking back, I'm no longer sure it was such a good idea. She stopped appearing to be herself, and perhaps this was the first visual clue of the dementia, and total loss of self, which was to come.

So my mother never wrestled with intractable problems as she stood hesitating in front of a rail of clothes. Can you wear a leather biker jacket at fifty? And what about a floral tea dress? Jeans? How much cleavage is it permissible to show? What about the matter of covering the arms? With puff sleeves? (No, Joan Burstein told me, *no* puff sleeves.)

There is a ghastly poem which menopausal women seem to like, or their younger friends think they might like, in which a woman promises that in old age she will wear purple, and a clashing red hat, an ensemble that does not suit her. If it doesn't suit you, why wear it? When I am an old woman I don't want to be a mad old biddy in mismatched clothes, mumbling in the street in her house slippers. I want to be Joan Burstein in a Marni dress with a spectacular necklace a friend brought her back from India and a cream python Fendi bag. Or Catherine Hill in Christian Lacroix. Or either of the two stylish matriarchs tottering across the lobby of the Carlyle in Manhattan, holding on to each other's arms for fear of osteoarthritic breakages, each in a little black suit and patent high heels. Or the very old woman I saw at the Paris shows in 2002 who, in the company of a young boy, was in head-to-toe combats and copper earrings the size of side plates.

Between the right of women to wear what the hell they like at any age they like (the feminist insistence on not being told what to do) and the virtues of common sense, style, and taste, there is a narrow, stony path, and it is this path that one should try to navigate. For Catherine Hill, sitting in Starbucks at eleven in the morning in her black jeans, rapper's long chain, and John Galliano denim jacket with mink collar, is not mutton dressed as lamb, but rather she has a sophisticated understanding of how to stretch style to its limit, including elements of that all-important soupçon of hot sauce added to the dish, vulgarity. Vulgarity contained within the formal outlines of couture.

༺༻

But those of us who don't have a doctorate in advanced styling learn the hard way how difficult it is to dress over the age of fifty. For some years I had been looking for a leather jacket, a jacket which was neither a coat nor a blazer, but one which fell to a certain exact point just at the top of the thighs. This grueling quest had taken me to some of the most extensive leather departments in the world, including the Galleries Lafayette in Paris, where I saw every conceivable type of leather jacket except the length I was looking for.

There was something about a leather jacket on a middle-aged woman that to me is both tough and chic; again, one feels that the middle-aged woman has earned the right to her leathers, to this second skin. Perhaps it makes a reference to her own leatheriness; all I know is that I like the look on other people and I wanted it for myself. Ideally I would wear it with jeans, boots, a cashmere sweater, and a really expensive handbag.

In the autumn of 2007, I finally found my jacket, and modestly enough it was from Marks & Spencer. It was a new chic take on the biker jacket, it had a waist, and I loved it. The triumph!

Until I read the words of the esteemed fashion writer Sarah Mower, who in itemizing the mutton moments older women were best to avoid, listed the biker jacket:

Everyone past the age of 40 needs a "mutton monitor." I belong to a tele-phonic kaffee klatch that does the job without the slightest risk of false flattery. In the case of black leather biker jackets—this winter's high street sell-out—there wouldn't be the minutest margin of a doubt. Should one of our number be tempted to revert to Suzy Quatro mode, she'd just have to be stopped. The rock chick mantle must always be passed to those in their twenties, fact. That means it's the property of the likes of Amy Wine-house. Even Kate Moss, moving up into her mid-thirties, will be pushing the mutton-button with that one any minute now.

I was crushed. Had I read these words before I got the jacket, I would have definitely left it on the rack. But now I had it, and couldn't wear it—or could I? I was no longer sure.

On my blog, a reader responded with fury and in kind:

It's just another example of the way women are manipulated, put down and even isolated from each other. Our whole fashion and beauty indus-try is based on guilt, shame and viciousness. Buy that leather jacket—and get the whip that goes with it so you can beat any sanctimonious naysayer who says you shouldn't (aren't entitled to) wear it!

Faced with this onslaught, Sarah Mower responded a couple of weeks later in print:

Pretending to be 10 or 20 years younger than you are always shows. When it becomes truly desperate, people will catch their breath at the sight of you, only to let it out as a laugh behind your back. So all I was saying was this: dressing "younger" can actually make you look older, and absurd with it, so don't get caught out by accident.

Truly, 2007 has been a bad time for this. Though I'm averse to laying down laws, some of the people I've seen in girly above-the-knee dresses oughtn't have worn them—a point comically exacerbated by the addition of "on-trend" 6in-high wedges.

I don't care how skinny you are, or how toned your body: when the face-age doesn't match the dress-age, you look silly.

And, of course, she was quite right. The ghastly discrepancy between the age of the face and the body beneath it is one of the most depressing aspects of ageing. It reminds me of those women who, having taken HRT and got their mojo back, work a room at a party, flirting with every available man, irrespective of age, convinced that how they feel inside is how they appear to others. Usually while they are wearing a low-cut top revealing a large brown wrinkled bosom.

So what the hell do you wear? For when I look at those infrequent magazine features depicting how to look fabulous at any age, and get to me, my age, all I see are those styles despondently known as classic: the classic trousers, the classic trench coat, the classic shift dress, the classic pantsuit, the classic white shirt, the classic low-heeled Ferragamo shoes, and the classic Chanel 2.55 handbag.

I never see anyone wearing this gear in the old films I watch on the classic movie channel, TCM. I see Bette Davis in deep red lipstick, snarling.

I don't want to wear any of those things, for the straightforward reason that all of them look awful on me. Because I lack an inner frump, they sit on top of my body as if I were one of those children's paper dolls you cut out and then fold outfits onto at the shoulders with tabs. I look absolutely nothing like myself. Depicted on Bianca Jagger and Catherine Deneuve, these classics look sensational, but they look good not because these women are in their fifties or sixties, but because they happen to be the kind of style that suits them. And because, being ravishingly beautiful to begin with, they can wear a sack (clinched at the waist with a chocolate suede belt, with heels and a gold necklace) and look as if they were doing the runway for Yves Saint Laurent.

The classics guarantee my invisibility. They create an immediate dislocation between the inner and the outer self, because I am not a self-effacing person. There are times when one wants anonymity and there are ways to dress accordingly. The great travel writer Norman Lewis, who bought his suits at Savile Row, always wore the blandest trousers and drip-dry shirts when he set out on a journey, not for the sake of his laundry but so he could observe, unseen. He inveigled his way into tricky situations by appearing so harmless and innocuous that warlords, militias, and company goons would take him for a doddery old boy. This technique allowed him to bring back the untold story of the genocide of the Indians of the Brazilian rain forest.

But most of the time, I wish to be seen. I prefer it that my clothes express something of who I am, conceal as well as they are able my numerous flaws, are aesthetically pleasing, and demonstrate some understanding of style and current trends while not being in thrall to the fashion pages. For as the magazine editor Louise Chunn pointed out to me, "Getting old in the fashion world is not a very nice sight. Many of them look a bit tragic, a bit madwoman in the attic. They want to always be fashionable because they can't bear not to have the latest thing."

Ideally one would be what Simon Doonan calls a glamorous eccentric, one of those individuals who never follow fashion but completely ignore it, creating their own rules which exist solely for themselves alone, like Isabella Blow, who wore a lobster hat and much other craziness of her own devising. But to be a glamorous eccentric one requires not just glamour but also eccentricity, which is not a condition of being well-dressed, but an essential aspect of one's identity. I would not call myself eccentric. And glamorous eccentricity amounts to exhibitionism, like the activities of Doonan himself, who excitingly walked out of the lobby of his Greenwich Village apartment building on a Saturday afternoon dressed as Queen Elizabeth II attending a state banquet (only to have his doorman address him, as if he were attired in jeans and a John Deere cap: "Do you want your mail now, or when you come back?").

But I have come to think that while eccentricity does not suit all of us, glamour is a habit which can be acquired. Glamour is what characterized my mother's generation of middle-aged women, it is what makes the classic movies so original and absorbing to watch. It is glamour that gives the women their strength.

As a word, glamour only entered the English language at the end of the eighteenth century, coined by Sir Walter Scott who Anglicized "glamer," which had been in use in Low Scotch for around a century and which means, "the supposed influence of a charm on the eye, causing it to see objects differently from what they really are." Glamour has always been a mixture of magic and artifice, of the visual illusion. Glamour is spectacle, composed of equal parts dream, illusion, envy, emulation, sex appeal, fakery, and surface. It's always a performance.

The Hollywood stars of the 1940s—Bette Davis, Joan Crawford, Katharine Hepburn, Deborah Kerr—were middle-aged women playing middle-aged women, a phenomenon which has almost ceased to exist in present-day cinema. The old-fashioned "woman's picture," today demoted to the "chick flick," was often a melodrama, featuring a woman garbed in an Edith Head or Adrian evening gown on a cliff above a stormy black-and-white nighttime sea. By comparison, the juvenile leads seemed insipid.

Those of us born after the war grew up with this image of glamour in our heads. Glamour was associated with the artificial, with the high sheen of silk stockings, of face powder, the unseen underpinnings like the corset, Marilyn Monroe and Elizabeth Taylor's drawn-in beauty spot. You knew it was a production. The fashion that replaced it had nothing to do with glamour, it was all about youth, the revolt against the insincere, the artificial, the phony. It was the barely pubescent Twiggy, aged fifteen, with no hips or breasts, just pipestem legs, a blanked-out mouth covered with the same pancake foundation as her face, and doll-like eyelashes. Before Twiggy, models had strived to look like women. One of the very greatest, Dorian Leigh, did not begin her modeling career until she was twenty-seven. They looked middle-aged when they were still in their teens because fashion was about womanhood, not girlhood; the teenager was an invention of the 1950s.

I can think of nothing worse than to have been a middle-aged woman who loved fashion in the 1960s, because fashion hated middle-aged women. The clothes themselves were impossible: the little round-necked, sleeveless minidresses, cruelly exposing wobbling arms and thighs while covering up a well-developed bosom. The antagonism toward artifice made the black arts of makeup themselves a vivid symbol of ageing. The face needed to appear not to be wearing makeup at all, as a sign of youth and freshness.

Glamour went out with the garbage in the 1960s, along with all the rules about how to dress. Dressiness itself was middle-aged. Whatever you might have learned from your mother to see you into the next six decades was rejected as out-of-date information. They wore those diamonds and strings of pearls for a reason: to reflect light up toward the lined face.

Creatures of surface, mirrors have a simple story to tell us and fail over and over again to reflect back the gift of our inner beauty and hard-won wisdom. Forty years later, we have had to relearn the black arts of artifice. So I have come to reject the classic charms of the beige trench coat in favor of glamour, or at least clothes with attitude. Not the girlish charms of the sprigged tea dress or jeans, but old-school in-your-face, sock-it-to-me-Mamma high heels and a hint of cleavage.

To dress like a teenage girl in little dresses with tights is to court pity. To dress like a hip-hop star is to arouse interest and possibly fear. Rappers understand glamour. If you come from the ghetto, like my immigrant grandparents, you understand that getting out involves dressing the part. The flaunting of wealth, the love of labels—this essential vulgarity is a life force. And at sixty, God knows you need as much of that as you can get.

At sixteen and again at sixty you are at the age when you use clothes to discover new identities. To stand in front of the mirror and see a different person with each garment you put on: to explore all those possibilities, those various selves. Never go beige into that good night, there will be more than enough time for neutrals in the darkness of the grave.

Carried on their shoulders, a silent, immobile lady had entered the room, a lady of oakum and canvas, with a black wooden knob instead of a head. But when stood in the corner, between the door and the stove, that silent woman became mistress of the situation. Standing motionless in her corner, she supervised the girls' advances and wooings as they knelt before her, fitting fragments of a dress marked with white basting thread. They waited with attention, and patience on the silent idol, which was difficult to please. That moloch was inexorable as only a female moloch can be, and sent them back to work again and again, and they, thin and spindly, like wooden spools from which thread is unwound and as mobile, manipulated with noisy scissors into its colourful mass, whirred the sewing machine, treading its pedal with one cheap patent-leathered foot, while around them grew a heap of cuttings, of motley rags and pieces, like husks and chaff spat out by two fussy and prodigal parrots. The curved jaw of the scissors tapped open like the beaks of those exotic birds.

∽ BRUNO SCHULZ

EXPANDABLE WOMAN

SOME YEARS AGO, in a restaurant in Clerkenwell, an area of central London, I saw a fat man with the bristly blond head of a pink pig sitting at the next table. His thighs, in combat pants, oozed over the edge of his seat like ripe Camembert. Adoring, thin young acolytes hung on his every word, which he expressed loudly and with great confidence, throwing back his head and roaring.

"That," said my lunch companion, "is Alexander McQueen."

And a spasm of pure rage passed through me. For who the hell was this fat bastard to tell women that they were obese if they couldn't fit into a size 6 dress? I am tired of fat men telling women whose bones do not show through their skin that they should lay off the doughnuts. Karl Lagerfeld, fluttering behind his fan to hide the double chins, sweet Alber Elbaz, plump in his red bow tie, and McQueen—all fat men ordering the female population to starve so they can fit into their skinny frocks. McQueen, like Lagerfeld and Marc Jacobs, would later slim down with the assistance of the finest trainers money can buy and no obligation to prepare family meals three times a day. Indeed, Lagerfeld managed successfully to turn himself into his own corpse. But it is a funny thing that fashion, which makes all its own rules, should adhere to Wallis Simpson's adage that you can never be too rich or too thin when it comes to being the customer, but merely that you can never be too rich when it comes to being the designer.

Here we all are, in our bodies. We have to wear something. If you have nothing, the very last nothing you will have is the clothes on your back. A starving man will sit on the pavement begging for food and a thousand people will pass him by and give him nothing. A naked man will be hauled off to the police station in a blanket.

While there are always the types who gaze blurrily at themselves in the fogged bathroom mirror for a moment in the morning and then put on whatever is clean, most people, almost all women, like clothes which, in a very simple phrase, *fit and flatter*. And will suffer abject humiliations trying to find such garments, because they have little choice otherwise but to stay at home in a black sack.

The world of clothes and the world of nakedness are so far apart that the body clothed and the body unclothed often seem like the meeting of a cheetah and a slowworm, each staring in animal incomprehension at the other. There is great shame in nakedness. Once this shame derived from sex, from Eve's primal realization that she was naked. Now it comes from the deep anxiety and despair that we do not resemble the perfectly toned, tanned, and airbrushed creatures we see in magazines. We are ashamed that we can't fit into the smallest size of clothes that they sell in the shop. We are deeply ashamed that our bodies are so immense and whalelike. My sister, who is size 10, in Le Bon Marché in Paris was unable to fit one limb into the leg of a pair of Balenciaga trousers. The saleswoman snickered.

Coming, as I do, from a family of Polish and Russian peasants, bred for bearing ten children and murdering hens with our bare hands, I have wrists that are too large for some bracelets and ankles that would make Christian Louboutin weep tears of horror over his cobbler's last. I was thin for four days in 1978, when I ate once a day and only consumed sashimi. My father was fat. A big man. My mother was petite, but two caesarean sections gave her that jelly belly which she felt by necessity had to be held in by the rubberized panties called a roll-on, or girdle.

The shame that lies beneath our clothes contaminates everything. Deep inside we feel fat or shriveled, our boobs are too small or they droop too low, our bellies are distended or they lack the muscles which we see displayed on the front of magazines like *Men's Health*. The flesh beneath the arms waves about in the breeze. The pubic hair spreads rapidly and abundantly across the thighs. Bunions. Ingrown toenails. Wrinkled necks. Dimpled knees. A withered décolletage. The flaws in our body, flaws never seen by anyone but ourselves, and our very nearest and dearest if we can help it, are considered to be a kind of disgrace. And are so keenly felt that they are held up to the most intensive scrutiny, which somehow evades the considerable drawbacks in our characters—a nasty temper, the tendency to take a drink too often, passivity, lack of courage, laziness, recklessness. The magazines are full of photos sneering at celebrities' bodies, but far fewer sneering at their bad manners and monomania. Because the celebrities know when they see the unflattering pictures that they have been caught dead to rights, they are too insecure to disagree.

If you go to the swimming pool, what you will notice, especially if you enter the sauna, is that there is no common shape. There are tall women with short waists. Long-torsoed women with stumpy legs. Women with bodies like bullets balanced on graceful, lean thighs and calves. Women with large breasts and flat buttocks. Women with enormous butts and tiny waists. Little boylike women who seem to have bypassed adolescence and never acquired a curve, just tiny little breasts that are small swellings beneath the nipples. Women whose breasts hang like empty receptacles, halfway to their knees. And each of them is existentially alone in her knowledge of her limitations. They eye each other, appraising and envying. Occasionally a woman comes in with what appears to be a perfect body. And no one notices.

When we set out to buy new clothes we are taking along not only an interest in fashion, but also an internal hell of insecurity or self-loathing about what it is to be clothed, and because we're buying clothes, not putting ourselves up for the Nobel Prize, it is the body and its horrible failings that matter. It's really irrelevant that you are a wonderful mother and wife, or that you have a doctorate in particle physics. If the clothes in the shops don't fit you, then none of your accomplishments will help.

In an interview, the British designer Betty Jackson (who, by the way, and I would not mention this normally but we're talking about the limitations of the body, has only one leg) told the *Daily Telegraph*: "I still think that clothes look better on thin people. I'm sorry, that's the truth. They look better in a size eight and ten than they do in a 16 and 18."

From the point of view of the designer, the clothes are, of course, the point. You dream of creating amazing things and sending them down the catwalk and making people want to buy them. Fashion is a visual aesthetic. It's concerned wholly and entirely with how things look. The designer is thinking about fabric and drape and tailoring and color and, above all, innovation, newness, modernity. Inside designers' creative brains teem new thoughts about what people should wear.

Pity the poor designer who must see his clothes degraded by proximity to the ordinary human body. A great chef slaves for hours in boiling conditions to create his signature dish, the pinnacle of his creative powers, and then someone who is merely hungry comes along and eats it.

The great couturier does not consider it his or her business to make the average woman who might wear his clothes look better, in part because average women are not his customer.

So we enter the shop in a simmering cauldron of insecurity. We want clothes that make us look fabulous. We know, minutely, our bodies' terrible deficiencies, those sagging stomachs and pealike breasts. Looking in the mirror at a tight torso swathed in bulging fabric or a drooping empty bodice, we see our faults are clearly on display.

It is pointless to argue, as a means of boosting our self-esteem, that in other cultures and ages fat women were admired; we live in the age we live in. To be transported back to an era where the heavy-joweled lady was the acme of fashionable perfection would be to accept all that goes along with that status: a lack of sanitation and death in childbirth. No thank you.

With wealth and prosperity comes the admiration for thinness. The visual image of women gets thinner and thinner, while actual women grow larger and heavier. The models are fifteen years old. The gap between who you want to look like and what, realistically, you are capable of looking like expands, so you feel you are staring across a howling gully, screaming fruitlessly, "I want!"

And the answer for many women is simply to give up. To regard clothes as camouflage. To wear tracksuits. Because there do not seem to be any alternatives, when shopping for clothes is so hard and painful and upsetting. Because you *cannot find anything to buy*.

This, to me, is the sheer strangeness of the fashion industry, compared with, say, a car dealer, who will sell you a car even if you don't hold a license as long as your credit is good.

The designers do not want fat women's money. They do not want fat women wearing their clothes. For they deal in the beautiful, and as long as fat women are regarded as ugly (as so many designers do regard them), then fashion must be what the other arts are, elitist, nondemocratic branches of the creative industries, and not at all a business which is to do with dressing women as well as they can be dressed whatever their flaws.

Fashion turns its back on its very subject. I don't mean the clothes that are sold in high street shops: they are not originating fashion, they're copying fashion, watering it down so we can wear it. By "we" I mean women who can't afford Alexander McQueen or Lanvin or Chanel. But what of those who can? Or who are, like Mrs. Harris in Paul Gallico's novel, prepared to blow their life's savings on a Dior dress? They can't, unless they fit the rigid demarcations of fashion's sizings.

So let's be clear about what fashion is (or is not): it is not a desire by designers to dress the body, it's the dream of a beautiful object, the craft process to make it, and its eventual display on the best possible canvas: the tallest and thinnest and youngest human form available. If five-year-old children came in six-foot-tall versions, you can be certain that the designers would be sending them out on the catwalks.

This disconnect leads to all the pain and humiliation of shopping. We are each of us on our own in the hunt for those clothes which *fit and flatter*. The heartbreak inside the changing room is the jeans that sag in the seat or have a rise which is too short.

We want fashion to be in our service, in the service of the human race; to fulfill our dreams of disguising our numerous imperfections. It isn't. And the fat man with the thighs oozing off the chair in the restaurant in Clerkenwell isn't interested in our longing to be made beautiful. He's interested in what goes on inside his own head and how to make it real. His own fatness is beside the point.

That is fashion. It isn't, you see, about us.

"All you have to do is to knock the heels together three times and command the shoes to carry you wherever you wish to go."

"If that is so," said the child joyfully, "I will ask them to carry me back to Kansas at once."

L. FRANK BAUM

FOOT-BINDING AND OTHER MODERN FORMS OF TORTURE

SOMETHING HAS HAPPENED to shoes. I can't walk in them. What is their purpose if they are not designed for walking? Is this not the function of these shoes? No, the function of the shoe is to fulfill desires. I didn't know that shoes were supposed to be love objects until I watched, from beginning to end over the course of several years, *Sex and the City*, which taught me the name Manolo Blahnik and that a girl could never have too many shoes. Because shoes are beauty, because shoes make a woman desirable, because shoes are love objects in themselves, because shoes give a woman self-confidence, because they are small sculptures in leather and metal. Because the feet are the part of the body farthest away from the brain.

I do not claim to have been a wearer of sturdy, sensible shoes until corrupted by Carrie Bradshaw and her posse. I have had platforms, wedges, stilettos, and sling-backs. Shoes with pointed toes, round toes, and square toes. A pair of towering espadrille wedges in harlequin colors. Fuchsia velvet embroidered and jeweled mules. My dearly beloved and long departed pink suede wedges. My red suede stilettos. My turquoise leather platform boots from the 1970s glam-rock era. My new Dolce & Gabbana black patent four-inch heels. Lovely, lovely shoes, but with the exception of the pink suede wedges I have never been in love with any of them; they have not inspired me with the same passion as, say, my cream patent Anya Hindmarch handbag.

I wonder when it became all about shoes. I wonder if women were nuts about shoes and *Sex and the City* merely revealed this hitherto unreported infatuation, or if it was *Sex and the City* which ignited the craze. When did shoes get more fabulous than a dress? And why am I sounding like Carrie Bradshaw, with all the questions, already?

Recently I have started to hate and fear shoes. I am afraid of shopping for them, which has become a distressing and difficult experience requiring physical endurance, chutzpah, and the ability to swallow large amounts of humiliation and disappointment. Shopping for shoes is one expedition after which I am increasingly destined to return home empty-handed. This is because I can't find shoes I can walk in. There is a name for the shoes they sell now—they are called car-to-bar shoes. You only have to navigate a little distance, the uneven terrain between the taxi and the entrance to your destination, a few tottering feet, before you subside onto a barstool and cross your legs in their shimmering 7-denier panty hose, raise a cocktail to your lips, and start to attract men. Fabulous idea, but not actually "relevant to my own personal experience," as the amateur critics say in book clubs.

For when I go out by taxi, it is to a party, where I have to stand for three hours, or to a restaurant, where my feet are hidden under the tablecloth. So what is the point of these fabulous, unwearable shoes? And why is there nothing else available in the shops but thin-soled ballerina flats which send pavement shock waves up my spinal column, or the shapeless pieces of dead sheep called UGGs, and Crocs, or luridly colored molded plastic boats designed to be worn while cleaning out the algae from ponds?

◌◌◌

The saying "Only the rich can afford cheap shoes" made sense because without protection to the feet, life as we know it is insupportable. At the bottom of this was the principle that things of quality last and badly made things don't, and when it comes to what you wear on your feet, you can't afford to cut corners or you'll find yourself hobbling about. You cannot walk, but more important, you can't run away without good shoes, and over several generations running away was more or less a constant in my family's history.

In one of the most memorable passages in *The Truce*, Primo Levi's account of his journey home from Auschwitz to Turin after the liberation, he describes his traveling companion, whom he calls The Greek (a native of Salonica), who contemptuously eyes Levi's weird shoes, the soles of which had become unstitched after only twenty minutes of walking:

> *"How old are you?"*
> *"Twenty-five," I replied.*
> *"What do you do?"*
> *"I'm a chemist."*
> *"Then you're a fool," he said calmly. "A man who has no shoes is a fool."*
>
> *He was a great Greek. Few times in my life, before or after, have I felt such concrete wisdom weigh upon me. There was little to say in reply. The validity of the argument was manifest, plain: the two shapeless pieces of trash on my feet, and the two shining marvels on his.*

Since reading this passage, many years ago, I have never completely forgotten its fundamental message. That without sustainable footwear we are pitiful creatures. Proper shoes are fundamental to our survival. But some kind of backflip has taken place, for women, at least, so that walking and footwear have broken free of what you might think of as a welded-shut connection which not even Charles Atlas could rip apart. But fashion designers have.

I am disturbed by the idea that I am limiting my capacity to move around. The pain of uncomfortable shoes, like a toothache, is never localized. It radiates through the body. I do not see men wearing absurd shoes. I do not see women attaching lustful thoughts to men's footwear. I notice that when men become completely obsessed with shoes, they are sports shoes. They have taken shoes you can run in and turned them into fashion items. How clever.

Very strange are old shoes, the shoes they wore before the twentieth century. The further back you go in time, the more they resemble winklepickers, those late-1950s teddy boy shoes with long pointed toes. Until the beginning of the twentieth century, fashionable shoes made for upper-class women were silk and satin, not leather, and their decorative qualities were enhanced by jeweled buckles (for both men and women). They were made of silk because women did not walk in the streets unless they were laborers, the wives of small tradesmen, or prostitutes, and if they did they wore sturdy leather boots. This began to change when women's lives changed. The Victoria and Albert Museum has in its collection a pair of Edwardian red leather shoes with a low curved heel, pointed toe, and lacings of silk ribbons. The museum's curator suggests that the style indicates the growing independence of women, who wanted fashionable shoes in which they could walk around town, in and out of the department stores, which were the palaces in which they were given the independence from the need for a chaperone.

Three pairs of beautiful kidskin dancing shoes from 1925, also from the collection, sit above a Louis heel, sturdier than the scaled-down stiletto kitten heel of forty years later, and in order to aid the fancy footwork of the Charleston and Black Bottom, they stay attached to the feet with T-bars across the instep.

Shoes remain wearable through the 1930s, with high but sturdy heels and rounded toes. Often they stay in place with ankle straps. In 1936 the shoe designer Salvatore Ferragamo invented the wedge heel and the modern platform. Faced with a shortage of leather, he took wood and Sardinian cork to make a platform sole and attached the shoe to the foot with cellophane straps. Although the wedge looked clumsy, it was excellent for walking and withstood wear and tear.

Platform soles gave women height, and during the war they balanced the square shoulders of a military physique. Both the wedge and the platform were the default shoe of wartime—you could run, fast, to the air-raid shelters in them, and dance the lindy hop. In France, during the occupation, wooden wedges were the only option available.

But you cannot wear wedges with the New Look, the petite, feminine silhouette. A great deal has been written about what happened to women during and after the war: the emancipation of women for war work and the sudden slamming of doors in faces as men returned home to take back the jobs that women had done in their place. It is not possible to make any sense of fashion—which is so overwhelmingly concerned with women's lives, what equality they do and do not have—in a vacuum which excludes feminism. The great changes in clothing have all come about because what women did and thought and felt changed. Every major alteration in fashion is always accompanied by an advance or retreat in social freedom.

Dior's New Look, which produced some of the most beautiful clothes ever made, the most ravishing dresses of the twentieth century which light up that portion of the brain concerned with visual and sensual pleasure, was agony to wear. The tight corsetry, pinching the waist in to an excruciating hand span made more obvious by attaching a peplum—artificial hips made of padded cloth—forced women to shorten their actual steps.

The shoes which were gradually developed by Roger Vivier to add proportion to the flowerlike silhouette of the New Look were as fragile as the women who wore them appeared to be. The tall, thin heels of the stiletto transmitted a large amount of force in a small area, and had to be strengthened by a metal rod and a metal or hard plastic tip. The great pressure transmitted through such a heel (greater than that exerted by an elephant standing on one foot, apparently) alters the posture, causing the hips sexily to sway out.

Oh, how I wanted those toe-crunching stilettos. Graduating from children's sandals to unbearable shoes was how you knew you had become a woman. The first stilettos were as much a rite of passage as a boy's first razor. Nicholson Baker points out that "Shoes are the first adult machines we are given to master." I understood that I had to learn to walk in stilettos in the same way as I had already clumsily, and with a great deal of falling over, eventually managed to propel myself across an ice rink on a pair of thin steel blades.

You practiced walking in your mother's shoes. I have a very clear memory of myself and another girl raiding our mothers' wardrobes at the age of six or seven and donning dresses that trailed around our ankles in the dust and our mothers' heels, which clomped along the road until we fell over, unable to manage the tricky balancing act of this enormous elevation.

There is a moment of transition when you know you are nearly ready and you nag: "Can I have stilettos yet?" "Not until you're fifteen." But fifteen was years away—we'd all be dead by the atom bomb by the time we reached fifteen. Girls of fifteen were aloof creatures in Max Factor pancake foundation, coral lipstick, and mascara which came in a small cake which you spat on and then vigorously rubbed a brush along to pick up its spittled surface.

But when I reached the "almost there" mark, when I came to be fourteen, there were no more stilettos. They had gone out of fashion. Dior's look, the womanly unapproachable sophisticate, was gone. It was replaced by the teenage girl in the little minidress and round-toed, low-heeled shoes—i.e., me. I was exactly of the moment. And as a consequence I never learned to walk in difficult shoes, I never endured the pain of crippling footwear and rose above it, because discomfort was included, it was what happened to you when you grew up and joined the human race. You accepted that your toes would be crushed into points and your heels would wobble about on unstable spikes.

I longed for stilettos to make a reappearance. I felt I had missed out on the true test of womanhood. And when they did, it was too late: too late for me.

So I have found myself, decades later, confronted with hellish shoes, shoes that are gorgeous to look at but make no concessions whatsoever to my having a life. I have started to wonder if this self-mutilation isn't linked with a general desire to hobble women.

From the tenth century to the beginning of the twentieth century, the feet of infant Chinese girls were wrapped tightly in bandages. Inside the cloth, instead of growing, the bones of the toes broke and became deformed. Swaddled in their tight wrapper, the child experienced intense pain in feet which were never to grow any longer than four to six inches. By adulthood, the girl's foot would be prone to infection, paralysis, and muscular atrophy. The ball of the foot would fold directly into the heel; the toenails continued to grow, eventually curling into the skin leading to flesh rotting away, and sometimes a toe itself would drop off. After three years of foot binding, by the time the child was around seven, the foot was more or less dead and the child walked about in the stench of her own rotting flesh. The pain would last for the rest of her life.

The ideal this barbaric practice was trying to achieve was the lotus gait, the appearance that a grown woman when she walked was "skimming over the top of golden lilies."

There are many gruesome practices still in use today: clitorectomy; inserting bags of artificial substances into your chest; pumping collagen into your lips; needling toxins into your forehead; the Brazilian wax. When I see the beautiful shoes in the shops, I cannot help but think of the forced crippling of Chinese women for a millennium. We are complicit, as the mothers of those Chinese girls were. And one is forced to wonder if there is something so threatening about women that periodically there needs to be a means of hobbling them—if that's the deeper meaning, or if it's more banal and straightforward, that it's just the normal fashion cycle.

For fashion does not do moderation. You have nice round-toed low-heeled shoes, and you must wear them with skirts which reach halfway up your thighs. You have ankle-grazing evening gowns, but they will be cut on the bias to reveal a fabric impression of every ripple and bump of your cellulite. And on and on. There is nothing easy or compassionate about style.

Pain and discomfort and distress are part of fashion. Fashion assaults our bodies and our emotions. "Give me shoes I can walk in!" I cry. And they offer me the revival of the loafer; in other words, how to make myself look short and fat.

And so I start to wonder if women are masochists: Are we actually the brain-dead dolts and bimbos which our superior brothers suggest? "It is only when the mind and character slumber that dress can be seen," sneered Ralph Waldo Emerson. "You cannot be fashionable and first rate," intoned Logan Pearsall Smith, the early twentieth-century essayist and author of nearly thirty works, most of which are out of print.

But then I remember that men get their teeth knocked out playing rugby, fall off mountains, run marathons, lift weights, and voluntarily sign up to be flown around the world to fight wars for the grand adventure of being shot at. Because pain is part of living, and pleasures without effort are cotton-candy confections, pallid and sickening.

It would be something if I could learn to live with sensible shoes. Lady traffic cop lace-ups, Doc Martens, T-bar children's sandals in primary-color leather, clogs. But to wear these shoes is to stand to one side from life (or life as I want to lead it, which doesn't involve a small farm in Wales, with obligatory rain over the low hills, and cluck-ing, shitting chickens). I want beautiful fashionable shoes which I can nonetheless walk in, and there is a permanent flaw in this unrequited wish. Of freedom and enchainment. "You must suffer to be beautiful," my mother told me, as metal rollers heated up against my scalp under a hot hood hairdryer. This suffering was borne without complaint as future generations would submit to the agony of the Botox needle.

There is a symbolic telling of this contradiction which has lived in my mind for many years, the Hans Christian Andersen fairy tale which relates the fate of the mermaid, daughter of the Sea King, who falls in love with a mortal prince.

On her fifteenth birthday her grandmother admits her into mer-womanhood, with advice which will reverberate throughout her short life:

> "Well, now, you are grown up," said the old dowager, her grandmother; "so you must let me adorn you like your other sisters"; and she placed a wreath of white lilies in her hair, and every flower leaf was half a pearl. Then the old lady ordered eight great oysters to attach themselves to the tail of the princess to show her high rank.
>
> "But they hurt me so," said the little mermaid.
>
> "Pride must suffer pain," replied the old lady.

Diving upward to the surface of the water, she saves the life of the handsome prince from drowning by shipwreck and, with the boldness of the free woman, kisses him. She goes to see the sea witch who tells her that to marry him she must give up both her beautiful voice and her tail. The sea witch tells her:

> ". . . I will prepare a draught for you, with which you must swim to land tomorrow before sunrise, and sit down on the shore and drink it. Your tail will then disappear, and shrink up into what mankind calls legs, and you will feel great pain, as if a sword were passing through you. But all who see

you will say that you are the prettiest little human being they ever saw. You will still have the same floating gracefulness of movement, and no dancer will ever tread so lightly; but at every step you take it will feel as if you were treading upon sharp knives, and that the blood must flow. If you will bear all this, I will help you."

To cut a long story short, the mermaid accepts, endures agony to win the love of her prince, but he is already besotted with his passion for the mermaid who saved his life, and, alas, she is no longer a mermaid. So he marries practically, to ensure dynastic connections, and the little mermaid is turned into sea foam, having won neither the prince nor immortality.

The mermaid's tragedy speaks volumes to me of these irreconcilable aspects of being female, our desire to give up a weightless freedom in exchange for the soul-enriching manacles of romantic life. We cannot accept that we continue to exist in our own element, governed by its own rules. We willingly walk on sharp knives. Accepting the pain is part of the human condition. I wish I could see a way out. I can't.

Take, if you must, this little bag of dreams
Unloose the cord, and they will wrap you round.

A GOOD HANDBAG
MAKES THE OUTFIT

WHICH WAS MY mother's motto. Outside my bedroom, arranged on the top of a bookcase containing the nonfiction section, is a row of her fabulous handbags. One of them, alas, barrel shaped and a burnished black patent, became so beaten up that it was no longer usable, but I could not bear to throw it away and so I sent it to the designer Anya Hindmarch with the vague hope that it might prove the inspiration for a new bag. Or failing that, that she would do the throwing away for me. In return, she sent me a tin of handbag-shaped iced cookies.

The other bags in my mother's collection include a silver sequinned evening bag with a rigid mother-of-pearl handle, a gold sequinned coin purse, another evening bag with a sylvan scene of the eighteenth century overprinted on silk with a black grosgrain back and a thin gold chain to carry it, and a completely flat rectangular black leather envelope from the 1960s by Charles Jourdan, in which a bunch of keys, a cell phone, or a wallet would make an unsightly bulge, so it can only be worn to keep your pocket handkerchief in it while your beau attends to the rest of reality. These are a *few* of my mother's bags.

Over the years I have added to the collection a couple of suede Fendi baguettes, one in red and one in purple; a black leather baguette-shaped Gucci day bag which I bought at the Gucci boutique on Capri while sequestered in temporary luxury, writing a novel; an oxblood leather and hair Luella bag with all the Luella bells and whistles—the straps and metal loops that make it like Fort Knox to get into—which I purchased at a *Vogue* sample sale in aid of Turkish earthquake relief, urged on by *Vogue*'s editor, Alexandra Shulman, who told me it was "a classic"; two Anya Hindmarch (my weakness) Carkers, one in cream leather, the other in brown mock croc, both designed for traveling; plus four other Anya Hindmarch bags, which I won't go into to avoid tedium, though one is black and gold patent and my favorite is cream patent with a chain handle; and a lot of other bags, like the Dolce & Gabbana green suede baguette I got in the Bloomingdale's sale and a Ferre which I ordered online from America with a huge discount but turned out to be no good (something about the structure made it look clumsy). Sadly I recently threw away two of my favorite bags: the Furla I bought at Selfridges' sale two days after the London bombings, which was caught in a heavy downpour in Budapest and the leather ruined; and the Fausto Santini bag I got at the Rue du Cherche-Midi in Paris, whose slim straps eventually broke because I put too much inside it. Which reminds me of a little shop on that street that no longer exists called Gingko, which made quilted nylon bags in jewel colors, and I have two.

I have nothing by either Chanel or Hermès—neither of the two great classic bags, the Chanel 2.55 or the Hermès Birkin, which starts at £3,500 (about $5,600). For this reason it cannot be said that I have a serious handbag collection. Looking at my bags, I sometimes feel that they are a library with no Shakespeare or Milton.

My collection long precedes the strange craze which grew up in the middle of this decade for the It bag and indeed was somewhat blighted by it, because as price inflation hit the handbag market, the bags I wanted soared out of my reach. I had thought it was enough to pay £200 (about $325) for a bag, and was startled to discover you could buy quite ordinary bags by Dior and Fendi for £400 ($650). And then it was £600 ($975), and then it was £800 ($1,300), and then the bags I admired cost over £1,000 ($1,600) and eventually there was the $100,000 handbag, as intended to be carried by Cate Blanchett at the 2007 Oscars, a Lana Marks bag in black alligator with a frame of 18-carat gold, white diamonds, and 35 carats of pavé black diamonds. Unfortunately it was stolen from her hotel room before she had even put a high-heeled foot on the red carpet.

The craze for It bags reminds me of seventeenth-century Dutch tulip fever, when trading in tulip bulbs turned into a form of economic hysteria. One bulb was bought with foodstuffs including a thousand pounds of cheese and two barrels of butter, plus a marriage bed with linens. Its equivalent cash value was the price of a large house.

The frame leather bag did not exist until the mid- to late nineteenth century. It is entirely a product of women's emancipation. Bags before then were made of silk, satin, fine chain. They were embroidered, beaded, and embellished, but they were not designed to carry much, and were usually worn within the home or for evening wear. Middle- and upper-class women did not need what we think of today as a handbag until they began to leave the house and walk abroad. The handbag is a necessity of city living, and of the freedom to be out and about, and of the emergence of makeup. When respectable women began to use lipstick and face powder which needed to be reapplied throughout the day, she had to have a handbag in which to carry these necessities. The bags made in leather by saddlery firms like Hermès had metal fastenings (to avoid theft while on the streets) and a compartmentalized interior with pockets for a fan, tickets, cosmetics, money, opera glasses, and cigarettes. For late-nineteenth-century women, the handbag must have seemed as revolutionary a gadget as the invention of the Sony Walkman. And it added an additional layer to the mystique of a woman: it was the depository of her secrets.

Katherine Mansfield in a short story called "The Escape," written in 1920, describes a frame handbag and its contents:

The little bag, with its shiny silvery jaws open, lay on her lap. He could see her powder-puff, her rouge stick, a bundle of letters, a phial of tiny black pills like seeds, a broken cigarette, a mirror, white ivory tablets with lists on them that had been heavily scored through. He thought: "In Egypt she would have been buried with these things."

The contents of a woman's bag, her paraphernalia, is as intimate as her dressing table or her lingerie drawer. Chanel designed her 2.55 bag with an inner zipped pocket beneath the flap to conceal her love letters. The bag carried by the working mother is the bag of worries, of large and small anxieties. In the working mother's bag is a Black-Berry and a bottle of Children's Tylenol. The bag carried by the single woman replaces the Children's Tylenol with condoms.

How you carry your bag goes in and out of fashion. The clutch, clamped under the arm, prohibits large gestures and is the bag for 1950s ladylike life. The wartime shoulder bag permits a woman to have her hands free for other more important matters. The gas mask box, slung across the chest, doubled up as a handbag. In 1935 *Vogue* advised that there was a new way of carrying a bag, no longer hooked over the arm but dangled on the hand by the handle: "We've already seen several smart women swinging them that way. A small point but it looks new. Try it."

By the time I was old enough for a handbag, in the 1960s, they had reverted to their eighteenth- and nineteenth-century predecessors, informal patchwork, embroidery, carpet, and ex-army bags, always carried over the shoulder, for there was nothing so bourgeois as a leather-frame handbag. Indeed there was something absurdly self-conscious about carrying a handbag at all, as if one was aping one's mother, for the frame bag was a grown-up accoutrement. Young girls did not carry powder and paint around with them, we fresh-faced innocent darlings. The frame bag had about it poise, certainty, and the possession of a wallet with sufficient amounts of cash, and possibly that new and frighteningly adult possession, the credit card.

Bags reemerge in the 1970s as the means by which working women were able to carry around their lives, but they had lost their frames and become large, soft, shapeless, and functional receptacles which closed with a zipper or snaps. The only two people observed to be carrying a frame handbag in the Britain of the 1980s were Queen Elizabeth and Margaret Thatcher. The prime minister's handbag: There was something thrillingly absurd about the conjunction; it was a superfluous feminine accessory, as if Mrs. Thatcher carried hers primarily to prove she was a woman, not a man, or a species of *vagina dentata*. And the bag itself, stiff and leathery, seemed in her hands to be a weapon of assault. To handbag. To clout your political enemies. To bash around the head. (Indeed I did this myself: I hit a man with my bag in 1988, outside the now defunct Lumiere Cinema on St. Martin's Lane, causing him to stumble and fall into the gutter—a fitting punishment for crimes I won't name here but would make you gasp if I did.)

There was something so ridiculous about the handbag that the way around it, the opposition to the monarchical or prime-ministerial bag, was a nylon satchel by Prada which you could buy from a blanket spread out on the pavement in Naples, sold by a thin African for a few quid. The first fakes.

But I was always carrying my mother's bags. The leather-framed bags she had bought in the 1950s were too heavy for her now deteriorating body. She got herself a little blue bag at Marks & Spencer, which she wore slung across her body and tightly clasped. She feared she was a perfect mugger's target, and she was. So the burnished patent, the crocodile, and the sequins were borne away by me, infatuated with their sophistication. The rebelliousness of my adolescence and twenties was always slightly undermined by my admiration for those *soignée* 1930s goddesses in Madame Grès draped dresses, and the femmes fatales and harridans of the silver screen, the melodramatic heroines of films noirs: Bette Davis, Joan Crawford, Rita Hayworth, Mary Astor, and Veronica Lake. However old they were, whatever role they played, they always acted and looked like thirty-five. The age of experience. If carrying a handbag was a mark of being a grown-up, then my bags were the means by which I ascended that ladder into adult life.

And, of course, they always have them in your size, and they always fit, which is the sheer beauty of a bag, with no fruitless schlepping from store to store, no miserable trying on. No anguished looks in the mirror. You are never too young for a bag, there are no mutton-dressed-as-lamb issues. And genuinely a lifetime's purchase, as the row of my mother's bags attested. They could pass from one generation to the next, and I recently bought on eBay a chrome 1930s Art Deco evening bag which came with a mirror and spaces for lipstick and face powder. There is one just like it in the collection at the Victoria and Albert Museum.

I do not understand others' lack of interest in bags. They use the same one, day in, day out, usually black, occasionally brown. Its depressing practicality drags any outfit down to the lowest common denominator. It is the accessory equivalent of the graying bra and torn panties, except at least you can't see those. The dreary bag stands independent of the clothes it was supposed to go with, as if it is outside fashion and style and taste. Humdrum and yet absolutely essential.

When I occasionally raise the question of the boring bag, I receive the eye-rolling gaze of those who have transcended the lady-like matchy-matchy preoccupations of the ageing generation which needed to color-code their bags with their shoes and their shoes with their gloves. You could, they suggest, do without a bag altogether. You could use, instead, a leather or nylon backpack.

⁂

I thought I knew all about handbags. I believed I understood the importance of a bag and that my mother would be proud of my own collection. Yet nothing she had taught me could have been preparation for what came next. My mother bought bags because she liked the look of them, because they pleased her eye, were good quality, and were the right size for her. I bought bags because I, too, simply liked them. It did not concern me what name was on the bag, and though of course I would have loved a Chanel bag, and perhaps regret that I have never bought one, I considered the price too high for what, after all, was just a handbag.

And then suddenly, out of the blue, secretaries earning £14,000 (about $25,000) a year are buying £1,000 ($1,600) handbags because they have seen Keira Knightley carrying one in a photo in *Grazia* or *Heat*. Or Paris Hilton. Or Sienna Miller. Or Victoria Beckham. Or whatever half-forgotten starlet whose name you won't even recognize if you are reading this in ten years' time.

How did it happen? In her riveting book *Deluxe: How Luxury Lost Its Luster*, Dana Thomas, *Time*'s Paris fashion and culture correspondent, describes how Japan in the 1980s drove the demand for luxury goods. A new generation of single Japanese women with large disposable incomes went in search of European luxury brands both as status symbols and in the belief that names like Chanel, Hermès, and Vuitton were a guarantee of quality and craftsmanship. In a mass-market world of globalization there was a hunger for what were assumed to be the enduring qualities of goods whose value could be properly measured. It was like investing in gold during a period of high inflation.

As more and more women chased the exact same number of Hermès Birkin bags that the company had always produced, having not altered their production methods or increased the numbers of staff making them, the Hermès bag acquired a social and economic cachet which Prada or Chloé could not attain: money could not buy you these bags; you had to place your name on a waiting list. Though if you were a celebrity, then the bags were "gifted"—that is, they were sent free of charge. The rich and famous were not paying for the products that the poor and unknown were going into credit card debt to buy. And those with insider knowledge understood that you did not simply go into an

Hermès shop and ask to buy a bag and resignedly add your name to the four-year waiting list. You bought some scarves and wallets, you agreed to be put on the mailing list, and magically a bag would happen to arrive in-store a few days later.

The price of bags kept driving upward. The illusion was that an expensive bag was a lifetime's investment. You paid £1,000 ($1,600) now, but with careful use the bag would last until you were creaking across the lobby toward the afternoon tea cart at The Carlyle hotel. Hermès Birkin bags actually increased in value, so that a vintage bag from the 1980s was worth more than a bag purchased this week. Except that the longer the fever for new bags went on, the quicker the bags were discarded and rendered out of date. A Fendi baguette, the perfectly designed bag to wear securely under the shoulder in a bar in 2000, was as quaint as Victorian button boots by 2005. The Chloé Paddington, with its giant, useless padlock, was the symptom of a moment of excess lasting only months before it was also too embarrassing to carry.

Bags had acquired not only visible design identities, but names. As if you were buying not a bag but a personality alternative to your own. Carrying a Marc Jacobs Stam bag, you might as well be model Jessica Stam, after which it was named. The status bag, the visible display of an accessory everyone recognized, and knew the price of, was a sign of disposable income. For if you flaunt this season's It bag for $1,300, it means that you will have next season's It bag at $1,600, and so on. The bag is the woman's Rolex. But the bag is also the contemporary equivalent of what today's women do not have (don't want or don't dare leave the house in)—the mink, sable, or ocelot coat. Though this is not the case, I notice, in Italy, where in the winter women still wear fur.

If you were wearing throwaway fashion, the high street tunic dress that would be unwearable in a couple of months (not merely because it had fallen apart at the seams, which it would have done, but because it had passed from "must have" to eBay discard from early March to mid-June), then the bag was your status symbol, the one enduring emblem of your taste and income. If you could not afford an Yves Saint Laurent dress, you could buy a YSL Muse bag.

Yet as luxury became available to the mass market, the more luxury became devalued. It was a sign of status not to have *an* expensive bag, but a new expensive bag every season. The notion that luxury items endure was abolished. Status came from being able to discard luxury goods as if they were high street. What was left of real worth was either the difficult to obtain (the Hermès waiting list) or the ostentatiously, obtrusively flashy, such as Cate Blanchett's $100,000 stolen bag with the black pavé diamonds.

In Hong Kong, I dived off a muggy street, unable to catch my breath in the traffic fumes, my lungs contracting in a panic, and was taken up a flight of dingy stairs to an anonymous door with a bell. When the bell was rung and the door opened, a Chinese man eyed us, admitted us into an outer room, and reached into the sleeve of a red kimono hanging from a rail, in which there was a key on a long string, which he stretched across, snakelike, to a second door and unlocked it. I walked into a place my mother would have worshipped: a high temple of handbags.

It is difficult to describe the interior without resorting to Western stereotypes and clichés of the mysterious Orient (this was my first visit to China). Inside was a rackety, dirty room packed with fake bags, presided over by a frightening dragony Chinese woman sitting on a stool and her willowy young blond posh English assistant, who assured the customers that they were a reputable business. Except we all knew that the bags were fakes, these dozens of Chanel 2.55s which I was assured by the English girl were indistinguishable from the real thing for a fraction of the price. And they did seem to be much the same, not merely in the design, but in the stitching. And when I looked at the lesser bags, the Marc Jacobs in particular, it was very hard indeed to tell the difference, and it was later explained to me this was because they were made in the same factories, on the same production lines, often by the same workers, as the originals.

According to Dana Thomas, only Hermès, Chanel, and Vuitton make their bags. The notion that an Italian designer bag was hand crafted in Florence by a woman named Lucia with centuries of Italian bag-making skills in her fingers, who bicycled home across the Arno every lunchtime in her Prada jeans for pasta and a little light adultery, was an illusion deliberately fostered by the brands. A bag labeled MADE IN ITALY needed only to have had its handle attached in Europe, after the rest of the bag had been assembled in China.

In Hong Kong, every woman on the multitudinous streets seemed to be carrying a major designer bag. Were they real or fake? I had no idea; they carried them with the conviction of the young, fashionable woman who knows she is dressed to strike a certain impression, of uniform brand luxury. It was a devastating sight for the untidy, badly proportioned Englishwoman. The women on the streets had achieved that plateau of excellent taste the rest of us aspire to. I found it soothing, and extremely appealing to the eye. And terribly sad, too, for all individuality had been extinguished in the race for the calming plateaux of luxe and the self-assurance they bring. I did and did not want to be them. For they seemed to exist in a kind of morphine predeath, utterly calm and at peace with fashion. No worries. This season would be replaced by the next, easily and without ingenuity. You just knew what you were supposed to have and went out and got it.

On the way to the airport the following morning, leaving in a taxi before dawn, the harbor was alight, almost on fire, with the blaze from its water's-edge city. Not the glittering skyscrapers but the cranes in the docks loading the container ships heading out across the world, rolling across the waves with their cargoes of "European" luxury goods, made in Guangdong province, which abuts Hong Kong. I felt that I had been living in a dream world all this time, a hazy realm of self-delusion which believed Europe and America to be the center of things, and our geopolitical causes all that mattered.

At the airport I tried to buy a pair of Ferragamo shoes in the duty-free shop. But my feet, English size 6, Continental size 39, were half a size larger than the very largest they stocked. "Chinese women do not have such big feet," the saleswoman sneered (sneering is almost exclusively confined these days to salespeople and book reviewers).

When I returned home, I took all my mother's bags down from the shelf and reexamined them. They seemed to hold the scent not just of leather, but her perennial Elizabeth Arden Blue Grass perfume, which she had worn since the fifties, and my fingers could almost make out the faint impression of her little cotton handkerchiefs, folded in points, with a blue embroidered rose and her initials on the corner.

The bags had swung from her arm at so many dinner dances, family weddings, and bar mitzvahs, and I had seen her with them, in her prime, descending the lift in our hotel before stepping out onto the pavement, breathing the air of a foreign city, about to taste its unusual delights. I carried one of her bags at a party to celebrate *Vogue*'s ninetieth birthday. Kate Moss and her debauched beau swept in, in an atomic flash of paparazzi lights. My mother's spirit lingered in that room. Her taste, her certainty.

Our relationship was always difficult, particularly in the last years of her life, but the handbags became the true inheritance. You could not buy what they were made of, or what they contained. But it went beyond the bags she left me—it was the whole idea of how *a good handbag makes the outfit*, the understanding of a small but crucial element of style itself. A lesson which created my own bag collection, lacking, as it does the Shakespeare and Milton of Hermès and Chanel, but making up for those absences in its particularity and its sense of myself, scented with my perfume, Miller Harris Terre d'Iris, and dented with the slight impression of my house keys.

The charnel-house smell seemed to grow stronger and stronger till it pervaded the room and obliterated everything else. Finally Mrs Leighton said ... "[T]ake those clothes away ... I must either burn or bury them. They smell of Death; they are not Roland; they even seem to detract from his memory and spoil his glamour. I won't have anything more to do with them."

And indeed one could never imagine those things the same as those in which he had lived and walked. One couldn't believe anyone alive had been in them at all. ...

〜 VERA BRITTAIN

DEPTHS AND SURFACES:
FASHION AND CATASTROPHE

I WAS AT HOME in London. It was early afternoon and my sister, who was then living in Washington, D.C., rang me. I was to turn on CNN at once because a plane had crashed into the World Trade Center. And so I did and saw, a few minutes later, the second plane attack America, and sat, stunned, for the rest of the day, unable to move, impossible to turn away from the TV.

The next day, sorrow and anguish for those who had died, hearing the terrible messages the soon-to-be-dead had left on their loved ones' answering machines. And then deep horror, dread, and then nausea.

The skies were quiet and empty. London was unnaturally still. We didn't go out, we didn't attend parties, we were certain that we were next. We were always flinching at abrupt sounds. When the flights resumed over the city, we looked up in fear.

Like many British people, particularly those who love cities, I ♥ New York. New York was the place my hometown of Liverpool faced; on the other side of the Atlantic, we were the shadow of its greater vitality. Eleven million Americans are the descendants of those who set sail from Liverpool to the New World, leaving the Mersey and crossing the ocean to arrive at New York Harbor. So there is a natural affinity, and I like everything about the place and have always felt that I was wrongly born in England, when I so obviously was tailored out of the kind of material to be found in a doorman apartment building on the Upper West Side: facing Central Park but not too far from the New York Public Library.

The attack on New York, this attack on America itself, shocked and frightened me because I understood at once that it was an act whose significance in world events was going to be much like the assassination of Archduke Ferdinand in Sarajevo in 1914. Everything would change now. Still, on a human level, what interested me were the pictures of the people on the streets. When enormous catastrophe strikes, you are forcibly wrenched from your reality, yet in order to function the mind insists on reality being preserved more or less intact. The human system works hard to stop you from going mad, and part of the way it does this is to anchor you inside your own habits.

Among the memorable images were those observed at eye level. Of women fleeing the burning towers barefoot, holding their high-heeled shoes in their hands. Many of those who survived never wore high heels again, though one redoubtable woman, an inch under five feet, who worked for the FBI at Federal Plaza, told her family she would go on wearing her high heels if only so she could "cheerfully bury the heel of her shoes in the skulls of those responsible."

Much later, when there was enough distance, several years,

between the events of 9/11 and the writing of this book, I asked several Americans to describe to me what they saw that day, and how fashion had been affected by the declaration of war on their country.

A Brooklyn fine arts undergraduate who watched the conflagration from the other side of the East River remembers the men going to work that morning in button-down shirts and dark slacks. "French cuffs were popular that year, cuts were moving from sharp and minimal to frothy and romantic, but in the days immediately following there was a total breakdown of dress codes or standards. Everyone was wearing comfort clothes. I have never seen so many natives rocking I ♥ NY T-shirts. You didn't have to buy them, they were just giving them away on the streets. I saw people wearing sweatpants to the office, people grocery-shopping in their pajamas. It was the beginning of fall and a lot of people were wearing big loose sweaters. After the first few days, where we threw on anything clean and spent more time looking at missing-person flyers than in mirrors, people started to dress again."

Funerals, always fraught and distressing events, revealed differing ideas about dress codes: "I wore a conservative black suit when I gave the eulogy at the memorial service for my best friend who died on the first plane that crashed on 9/11. Another person who spoke at the memorial, a major film studio head no less, couldn't be bothered to wear a suit and tie."

After 9/11, clothing became a message. The message took two forms, overt symbolism and a form of defiance against catastrophe, the desire to go on as usual. The first route was taken by the mass of Americans who used their clothes to signal to the rest of the world their patriotism. The second, business as usual, was how the fashion industry regarded the catastrophe after the first unsettling days.

The American flag was incorporated into all forms of clothing. The Stars and Stripes were ubiquitous along every street, not only hung in windows and from flagpoles, or tacked on to fences, but emblazoned on T-shirts, pants, socks, underwear, jackets, sweatshirts, jewelry.

The last time the American flag had featured so prominently in dress was during the 1960s, as an ironic icon of the countercultural revolution, a desecration of the flag by turning it into a shirt or using it to patch a hole in the knee of a pair of jeans. A hippie in a bandanna made of the American flag had something to say about the war in Vietnam and about his generation; this time around, the flag was a statement of solidarity and defiance, not just in Middle America, but among cosmopolitans in New York and Los Angeles.

"The one thing I distinctly recall," one woman remembers, "is seeing so many fashions with American flags on them, and that lasted for about two years after 9/11. Prior to 9/11 Americans were not at all prone to wearing clothing with a flag on it other than the occasional Old Glory T-shirt babies wore on the Fourth of July. Flag imagery [became] so ubiquitous that it was the first thing an Icelandic friend of ours noticed when she came over shortly after on business. It was everywhere, and it was also the most common free download for companies that sell digitized machine embroidery designs into the home sewing market. The pattern companies got into it, too, and so did the fabric mills; Stars and Stripes fabric was sold in hundreds of patterns [for] everything from silk to polar fleece."

This message of patriotism answered a deep need to externalize the shock of what had happened, to show others how you felt and what you felt. You could donate money to the Red Cross, you could support your president and your troops, but on a day-to-day level, going to work, picking the kids up from school, or driving to the mall, the only way it was possible to register externally your feelings—sorrow, anger, resolve—was through the body, and the clothes put on it.

A conservative American woman recollects how suddenly the public mood changed: "So many illusions were shattered abruptly on that day that most Americans realized things would never be the same, not ever. As we watched the empty skies and waited for the next attack, a weird malaise drifted over the country. For the next year, it was as if everyone in the United States was clinically depressed. Naturally this would impact fashion, which seemed irrelevant. Red, white, and blue just seemed like what we wanted to wear, in our homes, on our cars, and on our lapels. I still have my rhinestone flag pin, suitable for all dressy patriotic events. We were truly wearing our hearts on our sleeves."

Flag fashion began to penetrate every dress code, even weddings: "My brother got married the following year and the bridesmaids wore bright flag red, the bride white, of course, and there was plenty of blue in the decorations. No flag imagery, no Stars and Stripes, but the meaning was obvious."

Even children were dressed in the flag: "Our local elementary school immediately dressed all students, without parents' knowledge or permission, in American eagle T-shirts with some kind of aggressive message. There was an assumption that putting propaganda on children would be welcome. And sadly in many families it was."

The flag became a form of uniform. As when hundreds of thousands left flowers, teddy bears, and messages in the royal parks after the death of Princess Diana, it was a moment of national collectivity when the desire to belong to a group, to share the feelings of the group, takes over. Individuality is no longer the point. This was not fashion in the way the industry understood it—no designer had put flags on the catwalk—it was a grassroots expression of common sentiment, as if the whole of America had the same thought at the same time and spoke of it aloud, through dress.

For some it was comforting, for others it was unnerving and even frightening. Not to wear the flag was to opt out, to grieve in private or even perhaps to think very different thoughts or to be suspected of complicity in the attacks. Arab-Americans and Muslims quickly understood that the displaying of the flag on their houses, in their cars, and on their clothing was a means of reassuring their neighbors that they were on the same side in the new war against terror (perhaps the first time a war has ever been declared against an abstract noun).

For outsiders, visiting or newly arrived in America, the experience of a country suddenly expressing its identity so forcibly through clothes must have caused great anxiety. A woman who had moved to the U.S. with her family eleven days before the attacks remembers a sequence of experiences: "We moved to the U.S. on September 1, 2001. I remember being in the stores midtown and being wowed by the variety, the amount and range of clothing available in New York. After September 11 it all seemed so excessive. All I thought about wearing was black, for the many funerals we attended, and for the depression we all felt. I still hate wearing black because I wore so much of it then.

"My son, too, was forced to wear some kind of Americana T-shirt, and for a frightened boy who wanted nothing more than to move home it wasn't good. I remember red, white, and blue ribbons and American flag pins being sold everywhere, on the streets, in malls, in stores, and by vendors outside the stores. And if you didn't wear one, some people were rather aggressive about why you weren't wearing one."

The factories which made the flag clothing (some in faraway China and India) had seized the public mood and flooded the market with cheap patriotic tops and pants. In fashion terms, they were a disaster, but like the handwritten poems attached to walls around Ground Zero, for some they communicated, in a necessarily limited way, otherwise inexpressible emotions.

For some, wearing the colors red, white, and blue came as a relief after so many funerals, so many black coats and dresses and suits and shoes. Red, white, and blue made you feel you were alive, and amid so much death and terror, the knowledge that you were breathing, that life was still worth living, that there were enemies to avenge or bring to justice were also part of the public mood.

Others viewed fashion as a means by which they could put back the clock, to where things were before that terrible morning: "One thing I remember very sharply. About one or two days after 9/11 (I was living in New York at the time), I was home because school had not reopened yet. I went in a drugstore. And bought a new nail polish. I think I was trying to convince myself that things were okay now. That I could again enjoy what made me smile before. It was almost a way of returning back to normal. I had always loved nail polish. And after I paid, the girl—and I remember her face as if it was today—told me: 'Have a nice day—if you can.' "

৩৩

The fashion industry did not respond by producing more elegant flag clothing than the cheap polyester T-shirts you could buy at Wal-Mart, though jewelers did sell ruby, sapphire, and diamond necklaces, brooches, earrings, and watches. The attack on America on September 11 happened at the start of Fashion Week, the first of the global autumn collections, which would move on to London, Paris, and Milan. Many international media outlets discovered that their sole correspondent in New York on that day, the eyewitnesses to this horror, was their fashion editor. America had sealed its air, land, and sea borders. It was impossible to get a newsperson in, while the fashion editor was unable to get out. Which of them knew the names Osama bin Laden or Al Qaeda, or the grievances against America in great swathes of the world—its shallow commercialism and deep-hatched wars?

Trapped, with nothing to do and no language or political context within which to express the enormity of what had just occurred, fashion suddenly had a mirror held up to itself. It saw for a second or two how others saw it, its own tawdriness and irrelevance. Fashion writing, a craft often practiced by those who are art school trained, is known not for having an adequate vocabulary to describe horror; indeed it perennially struggles to find words to convey what it already knows about, and if ever there was an indictment of the vacuity of the fashionable mind and its stubborn (occasionally heroic) insistence on ignoring reality, it was in the revelation that on September 11 the Yves Saint Laurent store on Madison Avenue, which had just taken delivery of its $2,500 purple silk gypsy peasant blouse with puff sleeves, received over forty calls to find out if they were still open and if the blouse was available.

The preoccupation of the industry was whether or not the shows should go ahead in defiance of dazed families still wandering around Ground Zero holding up photographs of the missing. All the remaining shows were canceled. The designers invited small groups of buyers and fashion editors into their studios. Tom Ford for Gucci had been planning a strip club feel with models descending from poles and lap-dancing the audience. "Obviously," he would later tell the *New York Times*, "I had to dilute that concept."

The industry wondered if the shows in Paris, London, and Milan would go ahead. It soon discovered that Europe took a tougher, more insouciant line on terrorism. If there had been fashion all through the Second World War, there was no need to abandon it now. As Ford remarked, "It was hard to think about [my] show, because after September 11, who cares? That was my mood in New York, but I felt very differently when I landed in London five days later. In Europe they're upset, but they lived through World War Two. They've had their share of horrific acts. And then I thought, This is not the moment to go into a dark, minimalist fog."

Ford was correct about the very different European attitude to acts of terrorism. The U.S. had never experienced an external attack on its own mainland, only homegrown terror. In London, five years later, when terrorists detonated bombs on the transport system, Oxford Street was as packed as ever two days later.

It was the last weekend of the Selfridges sale and I bought a Furla handbag I had had my eye on for several months. I had gone to Selfridges because I knew that the point of terrorism, its raison d'être, is to instill terror in you, to make you too afraid to leave the house, and I wasn't prepared to have my moods controlled remotely by a man in a cave in Afghanistan, or, as it turned out, four lads from Yorkshire, as captured on the CCTV screens walking into the underground station like a group of young eager urban ramblers, backpacks on their shoulders filled with explosives.

I went out that Saturday morning because I knew that if I didn't I might never be able to travel on the underground again and that my world would become so circumscribed that I would not be able to live in the city which had been my home for twenty-two years. Without the tube, I would be driven out of town.

The saleswoman and I had both come in on the same tube line, had both witnessed the unnerving outlines of the armed police with their assault rifles standing on the platform at Kings Cross as we slowed but didn't stop. Below, rescue workers were still trying to dig out from the deep tunnels the decomposing bodies of the dead. The people on the train were silent. I noticed that in one respect the bombers had not changed our way of life. We Londoners remained, as ever, imperturbably intent on avoiding eye contact and, God forbid, conversation.

So the saleswoman and I (she was young, and Muslim or Sikh or Hindu—I didn't ask) had this small moment of mutual comfort. She had been too frightened to come in to work that morning, her first day back after the attacks, but she was worried about losing her job. Once she got there, the older women in the store began to recollect the days in the 1970s when the IRA had bombed Oxford Street.

"They'd gone through it all before," she said. "And we've got an extra ten percent off today because it's the last weekend of the sales, so it's a good job you did come in, because you've got a fantastic bargain on that bag."

The scenes of complete normality on the streets of Central London two days after the attacks might be evidence of callousness, but I felt that there was a common if unspoken urge to reclaim some part of that mythical past, the blitz spirit. I had always wondered if it had actually been real at all, or government propaganda, pushed out in newsreels in which chirpy cockney sparrers smiled in the rubble. The famous photo of a milkman on his rounds through bombed-out streets turned out to have been staged: he wasn't even a real milkman. But in London in the days after the tube and bus bombings, I detected a powerful sense of unity—not necessarily political unity, but a feeling that London was just too vast a city to be terrorized. Physically it was too big. You could carry on, and most of us *did* carry on. Oxford Street, in that final weekend of the sales, looked just like Oxford Street on the final weekend of the sales. I'm glad it did.

But in New York, after 9/11, retail collapsed. Bergdorf Goodman, anticipating that people would stop shopping, canceled their orders with designers. Comme des Garçons and Christian Lacroix found that they had shipments of clothes on their way to America with no buyers. A month later, three days after the start of the Afghanistan war, the Paris collections commenced, some with X-ray machines and metal detectors at the entrance. Anna Wintour, editor of American *Vogue*, put in only a token appearance, and just three U.S. department stores—Barneys, Bloomingdales, and Henri Bendel—sent buyers.

At Vogue House in London, Alexandra Shulman was wrapping up the Christmas issue. She put a number of girls dressed in union jacks on the cover with the strapline "Fashion's Force. Britain's answer to America's flag fashion." What *Vogue* is about, she says, is escapism, into a world of the imagination and of clothes you will never wear, let alone own. And how can you be sober and serious about that? Whatever they did would be wrong, would offend. Fashion cannot fuse its own preoccupation with surfaces with what lies beneath.

Yet their profound understanding of surfaces allowed fashion magazines to unerringly alight on those images which somehow expressed what America felt. As one American noted: "For me, one of the images that lingers was printed in *InStyle* in (I believe) September 2002 inside the back cover. It was a photograph of the New York skyline, and where the Twin Towers should be, a hand holding up a postcard of the Twin Towers in exactly the right spot. Strange that a fashion magazine should so unerringly put its finger on my pulse. Unless that's what fashion does."

In the first full issue of British *Vogue* produced after 9/11, a number of women were asked how the attack on New York had changed their shopping habits. It was evident that despite the initial shock, those outside America had not really felt the impact on their own lives. Alice Rawsthorn, director of the Design Museum in London, replied:

> *"I can understand why people stopped shopping after the attacks. I popped into A La Mode the following weekend to pick up a Marc denim dress I'd ordered weeks before. When told it hadn't arrived because it was impossible to ship anything from New York, I felt very shallow."*

It was a common theme among the respondents, to use shopping as a form of anesthesia or escape. J. Maskrey, a jewelry designer, went on a spending spree:

> *"After it happened I shopped a lot. I bought a leather trilby from Dolce & Gabbana and an overnight bag from Louis Vuitton. It was shock. I thought, 'Is there any point in saving money?' It opened my mind, really; the best thing to do at a time like this was spend and enjoy. If I don't treat myself now, then when?"*

Joan Burstein took the long view:

> *"It's clear to me that everything has to go forward—that's the economy of the business—but we must go forward with caution. We should not stop enjoying clothes. Clothes make us look and feel good, which is very important. There are two schools of thought to cater to: those who enjoy fashion come what may, and those who play safe. For me, it's vital to have a light-hearted mood. I shall be buying less for Browns, I'm afraid, but more thought will go into buying for Spring and Summer. Women will indulge a little more on what they want, but their purchases will be careful ones. I remember the last war: we must go on."*

My own first response to the news of the attacks on America had been a stunned uncomprehending incredulity, the mind scrambling to take in what it was witnessing. And this stupefaction took hold because I really had not a clue about what was going on or who might have done this until I rang a friend, a photojournalist familiar with parts of the world which were unfamiliar shapes to me, on a map I did not look at, who talked about "maybe a syndicate put together in a training camp in Afghanistan." And when I asked him how he knew, he said he spent an hour a night on the Internet reading about this sort of thing, and anyone who didn't wasn't entitled to an opinion.

What I remember best were the arguments, the shrill condemnation not of the men on the planes, guiding them toward their targets, but of American foreign policy and, as often as not, of Americans. "You just have to watch *Friends*," someone said to me, "to see that Americans are foolish and shallow people." Politics and opinions forced themselves onto your attention. You were the recipients of other people's views whether you wanted to hear them or not. A textile designer who could explain to my untrained eye what makes cobalt blue overnight turned autodidact expert on the Middle East.

So when I looked at those first post-9/11 editions of *Vogue*, all I could think was that they didn't matter. That we had been sleepwalking through life; that we were this grotesquely fortunate generation, born after the war, who had enjoyed whole lives of peace and prosperity and boundless good fortune, without fear or threat. And looking at a row of handbags in Fenwick a month later, all I could think of were those women in Afghanistan walking like frightened blue ghosts in their burkas through the pitted streets of Kabul.

௸

Within a year or two of 9/11, with the revival of the economy, fashion returned with such force that the very power of consumer spending stunned even the industry itself. For while New York burned, the global superbrands like Zara, H&M, GAP, and Mango developed a method of copying catwalk trends and getting them into the shops within a week or two of the shows. Fashion entered a six-week cycle. The stock came in, and was on sale to clear the way for new garments, just over a month later. There were no longer clothes of the season, but of the month or even week.

The mood that had descended upon us—of understanding the fragility of life, the poverty and rage and humiliation of angry men in places we knew nothing of, the fear for our lives and the mourning of the dead—simply passed away. We adjusted to the new reality. The aftershock of 9/11 eventually gave way to a long, sustained consumer boom. Perhaps it could be explained by a mood of living for today, living in the moment, and those fashionistas interviewed by *Vogue* only a week or two after the atrocity had, with fashion's antennae, known what was coming. That when you have stared into the black depths, you don't long for more depths, but scramble to get back to the surface. Fashion's superficiality, all its inessential qualities of frivolity, decadence, carelessness, selfishness, and egotism were left unmarked by September 11.

Was it an indictment of the industry itself, and indeed of human nature? Should 9/11 have made us more sober people, forced to face up to the reality of poverty, inequality, and rage? Perhaps it should, but it didn't.

For fashion's point is the passage of time. Eventually the flags came down from the windows. The Stars and Stripes T-shirts now hang unworn in the wardrobe. The red, white, and blue pins gather dust in the jewel box. The fad for flag fashion passed, as, of course, fashion knew it would.

We went back to being what we are: people who enjoy pleasure. Whose inexhaustible supply of *I want* is the reason the shops exist. Who are now older than we were on that morning of September 11, and know that we must dress to suit the times. Our times.

The dead sit in their photograph frames, wearing what they wore the day of their wedding, or that afternoon at the beach, or caught napping on the sofa, or setting off to work on a cloudless blue morning having dressed for the last time.

This is how we remember them, in that shirt, that dress, a smiling bride or groom or university graduate. And we go on living, go on dressing. There is no choice.

CATHERINE HILL:
I AM FASHION

CATHERINE HILL WAS born in Košice, though she still calls it by its old Hungarian name, Kassa. The towns in Central and Eastern Europe slip about all over the map, unstable elements in a sea of geography, and the residents of Košice in the twentieth century could hardly sleep a wink without having to run down to the authorities every half hour to have their papers changed.

The small city had managed to slumber through a few centuries as part of Hungary until the end of the First World War and the dismembering of the old, rotting, cosmopolitan, polyglot Austro-Hungarian empire. The year after the war ended the downtrodden workers of Košice would enjoy three weeks in which they were citizens of the Slovak Soviet Republic, a proletarian puppet state of Hungary, until troops thundering down from Prague secured the city for Czechoslovakia, to be confirmed in writing by the Treaty of Trianon in 1920.

None of which matters to Catherine, because as far as she is concerned she is Hungarian, and Hungarian is her native tongue, not Czech or German and not even Yiddish, which was not spoken by the Hungarian-Jewish middle classes.

How big was Košice? A reasonable size, she says (according to the official census, the population was sixty-seven thousand in 1942 and about 11 percent of the population was Jewish). She describes a small city of industry and leisure, factories and cafés, not in the center of things, not a capital, but with enough urban life to stimulate an intelligent girl.

"All I know is I was able to walk to school, to the coffeehouses," Catherine recalls, "and I always remember that my father used to play chess and dominos and he taught me how to play." When dinner was ready, and her father was late, still hunched over his chessboard, her mother would tell her to run to the coffeehouses to fetch him, and she wondered why she had to do this, to interrupt her father's pleasure. "And I was so reluctant but I had to respect my mother's wishes because this was a family dinner, and my father always obeyed. So then we used to walk home and dinner was served. I have never been back to Košice, but I remember that we had such a cozy family, cozy in the way that in the winter in the living room there was a chimney and Mum used to roast chestnuts. When I was in Vienna two years ago, I saw the chestnut puree and I thought of those chestnuts."

She was, in those days, called Katerina Deutsch. Her mother came from a wealthy family, in the textile trade. She recalls her mother telling her how one day she went into a store—it might have been a shoe shop; Catherine doesn't quite remember—and saw her future husband working there. He was so handsome, she fell in love with him and had to marry him. Later the young couple opened a shop together designing and making duvets.

She was a great disciplinarian, Catherine's mother, "totally different from my father, more serious. Both of my parents were very handsome; he was an impeccable dresser, he loved looking at women in their high heels."

Clothes were of paramount significance to the Jewish family, almost as important as food. There were universal traditions, whether it was in Košice or Tunis or Salonica or Chicago or Manchester: you had to have (or give the appearance of having) new clothes for the high holidays, Rosh Hashanah and Yom Kippur in the autumn and Passover in the spring. I don't know what this says about your relationship with God, but it tells you a great deal about the desire to keep your head above water, and make sure your neighbors know you are doing all right. So Catherine received her new outfits for the religious festivals—the patent-leather shoes, the white socks, the new dress. God forbid you should go to the synagogue looking a mess.

After the synagogue the family would walk back for lunch to a religious home. She recalls the special dishes for Pesach, how her mother cleaned out the cupboards to prepare for the commemoration of the flight from Egypt, the twelve plagues, the slaying of the firstborn, the crossing of the Red Sea. Catherine loved soaking the matzoh in the milk for the morning breakfast. Her mother was a wonderful cook.

Sometimes she is flooded with a desire to go back to her hometown and see if she can find that place where her father was playing dominoes and chess. She remembers the courtyard of their apartment building, and the man who came to sharpen the scissors and knives, and the ice cream wagons. She uses the word *idyllic* to describe her childhood. "Yes," she says, "I think I had an idyllic life, I did not experience any death or sickness. I know that my mother did not have a mother and father, but my father had a grandmother and I used to go and visit her in the summer. Maybe it was a farm or a country house. I just know there was a beautiful huge kitchen and the dog was lying on the floor. My father's sister used to come and her daughter was also there and I used to take walks where the farmers were. The wheat was rising and the vegetables were growing—I had such freedom, I could go out at night, I could walk the streets, aged fourteen or fifteen, and nobody cared."

She went to other children's homes for birthday parties. She recalls standing by the window, looking out at the garden, and having a premonition that she would have a different life, that this, Košice, would not be her life. She was filled with curiosity and a sense of adventure. Wandering the streets of her town, she would look up at people's windows and wonder who lived there and what kind of lives they had. She knew then there was not just one way of existing.

1938. Košice is suddenly back in Hungary again and the government has entered into a marriage of convenience with the Third Reich.

No one in her family saw what was coming. They were Hungarians—

their government would not abandon the Jews. That was the depth of their faith in Hungary and their feeling that despite being Jews, slightly different, they *were* Hungarians. Yet what happened came up on them very fast, time speeding up, almost without the capacity for anyone to plan, or to escape. Suddenly Catherine was sewing yellow stars onto her clothes. What do your clothes say about you? They say *Jew*.

So it didn't much matter what they were sewn on to, a silk dress or a workman's shirt—the message was simple, brutal, had one meaning only. The cloth star was the most democratic form of clothing ever invented, apart from the Mao suit. Everyone who wore it was reduced to the same status, whatever the quality and tailoring of what it was attached to.

At home they talked about trying to get to Palestine. They had the money. Her father wanted to go but her mother believed in stability. And this was the only time Catherine would ever criticize her parents— for their faith that everything would be okay, the blunted instincts. (She remembered it, years later, when the Quebec separatists began their campaigns of bombings and kidnappings in Montreal, and she got out while she could.)

Attempting to take matters into her own hands, the teenager approached a man in the street whom she recognized as having once been a visitor at their house, an army officer.

"I said that I wanted to talk to him, and it was one of the most dangerous things I ever did because he was single and I was, I don't know, about fifteen, and he said, 'Well, come up, I'll talk to you.' And I remember sitting there with him and he looked at me, as a woman, as a sexual object. I said, 'We need some help, I think something is going to happen to the Jewish people.' But it was the way he looked at me. I got scared. I wanted him to help us, to advise us, but I saw there was a moment of danger and I left."

In 1944 the genocide of the Hungarian Jews began and the Jews of Slovakia were the first to be deported: all of Košice's twelve thousand

Jews were put on trains and taken first to the ghetto, then to the death camps.

The family were collected. They were packing, ready to leave for somewhere, to a labor camp, they hoped. What did they think *labor* meant? And what do you wear to face such an uncertain future? The urban deportees of the towns and the cities of Eastern and Central Europe had not held rough implements in their hands for generations. An important, even life-changing journey lay ahead of them, and their instincts were to dress up for the occasion.

Her father put on his suit, her mother wore a dress and sewed jewels into the hem of her clothes in case they needed money. All those Holocaust hems and linings, heavy with gold and precious stones, which did no one any good except the people who took them and gave nothing in return for the transaction.

Well, Catherine thought, we're going to have an adventure, we're going to travel, we're going to go to a work camp. It seems to her now inconceivable to have had this purity of mind.

For all her glances into the windows of the houses in her home-town, all those heads in the early evenings bent over a book or a piece of sewing under the amber glow of a fringed lamp, none of her curiosity had led her to the farthest reaches of the human imagination: what human nature is like and human pain.

Being herded together, urinating in public, the smell, not being able to breathe, to have no window and just a little water.

After around three days, the doors of the cattle car opened and she saw the SS men and the dogs. "That's the first time that I realized, well, this is not the kind of adventure that I am looking for."

And then everything moved very fast. She did not know where she was, she did not know that this was Auschwitz-Birkenau, that they are standing on the famous ramp where the trains pulled in, which unloaded the people in the nice clothes, with their suitcases full of red high-heeled shoes, and delivered them to the SS men who had taken into their own hands what had always been considered the prerogative of God: the power to decide who would live and who would die.

Catherine's mother was tall (as Catherine is today) and she had a very beautiful stature, but she was tired, losing her strength. Catherine looked around. Her father had now disappeared. She was holding her mother's hand.

"And I still don't know, I question myself about this all the time, how does a German person decide who goes left and who goes right? My mother was young and she could have been selected for labor, but I was holding her hand and I have several ideas that they saw this connection between us and they were so mean that they just wanted to separate us. Not only did they know that they were going to put someone in the gas chamber, but they wanted to hurt them by removing this family connection. They say the selection was random but there was more to it. The individual German person had so much hate and so much indoctrination from Hitler that they got satisfaction even before they killed you to separate the young, the children, from their mother. It was the worst thing in a human being that surfaced, because separating loved ones is the worst thing to do before you kill them.

"I looked at him square in his eyes and he looked at me, and he said, 'You go there,' and I said, 'No,' and he said, 'Yes,' and for one moment I was going to say, 'No, I'm going to go with my mother.' But I just let her hand go or she let my hand go, I really don't know. I would have to be hypnotized to remember it clearly. And in that moment I knew I was being selected to go the right way.

"I did not know at that time about the crematoriums. I did not find out until we went through the process of disrobing and shaving and the tattoo and until I went to the barracks. Some of the kapos were so eager—they were the Polish ones who had been there for many years and they were helping the Germans with the supervision. They told us immediately the truth. Were they warning us about the danger or were they just trying to tell us? 'Look at that smoke,' I remember one of them saying. 'You see where that smoke is rising? That's where they burn all the people.' I thought that person just wanted to scare me, he was nasty. I couldn't believe it because everything happened with such rapidity."

A teenage girl among strangers. She does not know where her father is, he has vanished. Her mother has gone straight to be gassed. She's entirely alone. (The clothes, by the way—the suits, the dresses, their hems weighted with gems, the furs, the dancing shoes—were collected in great piles, sorted through, and shipped back to Germany to clothe the civilian population, as a reward from Hitler for enduring the nighttime aerial bombardment of their cities. Thus the furs and cocktail frocks were once again paraded in the cafés and nightclubs while their former owners lay naked in mass graves. Nazi recycling.)

It's 1944. Catherine has spent all her life in a small Hungarian town among middle-class Jewish people. And now she sees something she has never witnessed before. The naked human body in all its alarming diversity. Hundreds, maybe thousands, of women of all shapes, all sizes. Women with young bodies, their breasts barely grown, their pubic hair appearing. Women with pendulous bosoms and drooping bellies. Fat women, skinny women. Women with long legs and women with short legs. Women with hips and women with no waists. Women with big bums and women with bums as flat as pancakes. They all stood shivering, naked, their heads shaved, their forearms inkily marked with an inked number, the infamous Auschwitz tattoo, an act carried out in no other camp.

It was at first the cruelty of it that struck Catherine—not only the cruelty of how they were herded, but the bareness of them all, how unprotected they were. The shame. Not just the sexual shame of nudity, but the shame a woman feels when her physical imperfections are brutally on display to strangers, outside in the open air, so everyone can see that what they have been trying to conceal beneath their clothes, by judicious dressing, is the figure that is no longer slim and youthful, or is just an awkward shape.

The only naked body Catherine had ever seen was her own, in the mirror. She had looked at herself, as girls do, and thought she was beautiful. Now she saw how the SS men viewed their bodies, their lechery. For they may have thought that they were dehumanizing their victims, by turning them into what they called *Stücke*, pieces, but you do not lust after a lump of wood. And perhaps, Catherine later thought, it was because the Hungarian Jews were the last transport—the last set of Jews they could find, having emptied out the rest of Europe, because there wasn't another country after the Hungarians—that they enjoyed the sight of the naked women all the more.

Years after, Catherine would understand how clothes are such security for us. It would have been different, she believes, if they had had their clothes—even if the Nazis had shaved their heads, but still left their clothes. She realizes now that for the rest of her life she has been clothing her own nakedness and the nakedness of the women she had seen in the camp. Even for those of us who have not experienced the horror of the camps, the desire for luxury, for beautiful clothes, can be the revenge against poverty and neglect and cruelty.

"I think they really got to you. Whoever devised the system, they got to the bareness of you—only animals wear their skin all the time. You see this imperfection of the bodies, the different shapes of breasts. It was the first time I realized there were different bodies from mine. I used to go to the Hungarian club, the swimming pool, I was surrounded by people who looked good and I used to think that everyone was beautiful, so this was a revelation—the belly hanging out, herded together naked, in silence. And it's the strangest thing, but I don't remember hearing cries. Everybody was anesthetized. I think it was the shock."

Growing up, Catherine had beautiful dark black hair. Her mother had braided her hair and put ribbons in it. Now she was bald.

She does not like baldness, even today. She does not like a bald man and she gets upset when she sees cancer patients whose hair has fallen out because of radiation treatment. When she sees baldness, she thinks of Auschwitz. Her hair had been shaved off, she was wearing a burlap uniform, a striped dress. And somehow she became extremely self-conscious about her appearance, especially her ears. Where, she wonders now, could she have seen a reflection of herself? Could there really have been a mirror? It seems unlikely. Maybe she just looked at other people and saw how they looked. She only remembers that she was acutely aware of her ears protruding, like donkey's ears or Clark Gable's ears, which she had particularly noticed when she went to see the film *Gone With the Wind*.

Early in the morning, roll call. The SS men counted you. It seemed idiotic. Where could you go, where could you escape? They could have let you stand there, but why the counting?

"So this striped thing, it was so long, and all I could think about was, My God, I'm so cold and I'm missing my hair, but my ears—I'm going to have to do something about this. I took the bottom of the dress and I tore a whole strip around and I rolled it and I put it on. I made a ribbon and I tied it, and I said, 'That's beautiful.' And I felt that my mother was tying my ribbons and it gave me a moment of content."

This act, the making of a ribbon which she tied in a bow and which covered her ears, a kind of hat, a form of millinery, was the decisive moment in what would be Catherine's long life. This human vanity, the caring about what she wore and how she appeared, the deep connection with her lost and murdered mother, who tied ribbons around her child's plaits, was her turning point in Auschwitz. And it makes you think about what those other women felt, that great incongruous mass of humanity, with nothing left of themselves but their skin and their pubic hair, shivering in the cold open air, watched by the mocking or indifferent or lascivious eyes of the guards, who themselves could never have seen so much naked female flesh.

Catherine was on the cusp. "I thought the German SS man would think it was defiance. We're standing in rows and we had hundreds of people, thousands, but everybody is bored and naturally you see there's one person standing there with this striped ribbon on her head. All I remember is that four or five people came. He had a stick or something and he motioned to one of the Gestapo women, or maybe it was a kapo came and got me, so I was standing in front him, and he said, 'What is this?' I did speak German—we used to have a German maid at home—but he had a Hungarian interpreter there, and he said, 'Ask her what's she's doing.' I explained to him in broken German that I just wanted to look pretty—that's the first thing I said. And that I was cold. And he started to laugh, a big laugh because he thought it was the biggest joke, which was lucky for me.

"So he gave instructions, I had to remove it. And all I know is that they put me to the kitchen to distribute soup to the inmates. The next day, one of the Polish women who worked in the kitchen said to me, 'You could have been killed, you can't do something like this!' But I didn't have to go to the gas chamber.

"Now I think about this, the intention was purely aesthetic and it satisfied me. I just acted from a natural urge, there was no goal. They could have got rid of me right there and then, but they could not take away my desire to be feminine, and a woman. And my dignity, even in the most degrading situation, when you're hungry. My father had had a wonderful sense of humor and I always tried to find positive things in the worst, so I always have this hope and desire that things will be okay."

For the next few months Catherine was shuttled between Auschwitz-Birkenau, the site of the mass genocide of Europe's Jews, and a subcamp where gangs were put to work repairing the railway line. In the deepest winter, often barefoot, she carried heavy rails in the snow, her feet frozen. The worst was the freezing of the feet, those parts of our body with the least pads of fat and the most exposure to hostile terrain. She remembers watching the struggle to live, the survival of the fittest, human nature at its best and its most degraded. You wonder if people were reduced to being little more than beasts or if they could escape into their memories? She talked once to an older woman, another inmate, in her thirties or forties, who told her what she most missed about her former life was cigarettes and sex.

Then one day, in January 1945, the Germans left. The gates of the camp were wide open, the Russian liberators of the Red Army had arrived. The women who survived walked out along the road and into the town on whose outskirts the death camp lay. All the houses were empty. Their inhabitants evacuated so fast that in one place Catherine and some other women found a teacup was still on the table. The Russians were going from house to house, looking for Germans. One of the other girls told her to go upstairs and close the door. She stayed in the closed room upstairs for a couple of hours. Why was she hiding? Because she was warned that if she looked pretty, the Russian soldiers might mistake her for a German and rape her.

It was the most ridiculous thing she had ever heard. She was bald. Who would want to rape her? But for women, that was the most frightening thing after the war, the fear of being raped, and as the records proved, a woman did not have to be young or attractive or well dressed to be attacked.

The survivors got on the trains, which were free and led them in the opposite direction, away from the camps. The journey home.

Catherine knew her mother had been gassed on that first day, when one of them had let go of the other's hand. Of the women on the transport that came in on the date she arrived at Auschwitz, most went straight to the gas chamber. She was extraordinarily lucky to have been sent to the right, the other direction, and to life. The fitter men, however, had been sent off to do slave labor and Catherine still had hopes that her father had survived, so she returned to Košice to try to find him. But when she finally reached home she learned that he had died of typhoid fever.

Catherine went to her old apartment and experienced the situation of Jews all over Europe returning to their houses and flats. They belonged now to someone else. Belonged perhaps not by law, but how could a teenage girl have the force to evict a family? You go home, and home is somewhere where a stranger shuts the door in your face.

What now? She could marry and start a new life, but after a few weeks she was certain that she did not want a relationship with another

survivor, that she would constantly be reliving "that Holocaust thing."
She liked one of the boys she met in Košice, but she had already made
up her mind about the future. The war was over and Europe was in
postconflict chaos, with vast populations crossing and recrossing the
Continent, refugees trying to find their way home, and demobbed soldiers heading in the opposite direction. By the time they reached their
destination, home might be a pile of leveled rubble or a locked door,
or under the administration of a foreign power.

The survivors were largely on their own in those first months.
There was no care, no counseling, no therapy for the people who had
just been liberated from the camps. The huge emotional and psychological trauma of the past, that fetid nightmare, was suppressed by the
need to survive from day to day in the present. And all Catherine could
think of was her desire to escape, to get out of Košice.

"I see this happen when you have a great love affair," she says, "and
the person rejects you and then the pain is so tremendous seeing that
person, you want to move somewhere else so you never have to see
them again."

One cousin was all that was left of what had once been a family, the
child of her mother's sister. They went to the uncle's house and, as
in a fairy tale, found gold hidden in the well in the garden, and with
her share of the money Catherine bought herself new clothes. She was
living by herself in a rooming house. Standing in front of the mirror, her hair just starting to grow, she looked at herself in a blouse she
thought was beautiful after all the months of that striped and filthy
burlap dress. Once again, pretty.

First she went to Prague with a boy, another survivor, and then she
met another man and went with him to Rome, traveling on his wife's
passport, her hair dyed red to imitate the physical description written
in the document. In Italy she was a refugee, a displaced person, and
the Joint (American Jewish Joint Distribution Committee) found her
a temporary home with an Italian family.

"I think my life started the day I arrived in Rome," Catherine says.

It was a city of joy, vibrant and alive in 1947, two years after the war. She walked along the Via Veneto and saw how handsome the men were, all the sexuality, the way they looked at her, the way they talked to her. The opulence of the emotions brought her back to life. Her hometown was a cemetery. No mood of celebration there. But in Rome there was a celebration, and the Americans from the Joint also got caught up in the atmosphere. Perhaps because of this, Catherine now feels, the people from the Joint did not really feel the pain of the Auschwitz survivor, but there was always the warmth and the empathy of the Italians. She felt a tremendous love from the family she lived with—especially the wife, Beatrice, and the daughter who was going to university.

"And in the beauty of Rome, the beauty I had had with my parents was also there, in Rome."

One day, on the eve of a party in Montreal in the early 1950s, when she was still married, Catherine used her husband's charge card to go to Holt Renfrew and buy a $500 Dior-under-license brown shantung taffeta dress. Early on in his career Christian Dior had found a way to get around the shocking numbers of fakes that were appearing in North America. He made deals with department stores, allowing them to sell licensed copies under their own labels. It was not Dior couture, but it was an attempt to limit the theft of intellectual property, the making of knockoffs by people in the rag trade who had managed to get admission to the Paris shows.

Five hundred dollars must have seemed a huge amount in the very early 1950s, and when Catherine came home with her Dior dress her husband hit the roof. How could she spend such a sum of money on a *dress*? She raged at him. He was treating her like a child, she said. But she went to the party in her new dress anyway and knew she was beautiful, and was happy.

"We were drinking champagne and this man came over to me. The dress had short sleeves and there was my Auschwitz number on my arm, and he asked me what it was. I said, 'Well, I never remember my telephone number so I just had it tattooed.' "

When they returned home that night, her husband had not forgotten his anger at her extravagance. Again he scolded her about the dress. But then he added another criticism. How could she say that thing about the number on her arm? Well, she said, she thought it was funny. What was she going to tell him? That she was in Auschwitz? For this was a time when no one talked about the black past and no one asked, either.

It was not only that her husband did not want her to talk about the number on her wrist to strangers, he wanted her to have it removed. And perhaps, she thought, this was a good idea. "I stood there and I said, Maybe it is right, that if the number will come out I won't remember what happened to me. I said to myself, I'd better do it."

But at the back of her mind was the thought that maybe her husband wanted her to have the tattoo removed not so she would forget the past, but because he was ashamed of her. That with the number on her arm she was a living reminder that once she had been a prisoner. And, of course, was a Jew.

She considers now that it was the act of someone who was still a victim, to have gone along with him and have it removed by a plastic surgeon, who did not do a particularly good job in those early years of cosmetic surgery. The faint scar is still there on her arm.

Catherine did not regret the little operation, the erasing of the past, until some years later when she was running her shop and a customer came in and undressed. She was gray haired but attractive. Her husband had died and she was dating a new man and she wanted a new dress.

"I said, 'You still have the number.' And she said, 'Well, don't you still have the number, Catherine?' I had had several newspaper articles written about me by then, about the tremendous taste I had and my shop and my success and the designers I had brought to the city, and they wrote that I survived Auschwitz. The city was surprised because nobody thought I was Jewish. So this woman said to me, 'I know you were in a camp because I read it in the paper.' And then I relived that moment when my husband told me to have it removed. I thought, My God, how could I do a thing like that?"

She can no longer remember her number. When it was removed, she wrote it down on a piece of paper, but it was lost. She still thinks it is a dilemma, what to do about those marks they left on her body.

"Yesterday I was thinking about revisiting Auschwitz," she said to me, "and I thought that maybe looking at your number every day may not be a good idea anyhow. So it's really a double-edged thing."

Many survivors of Auschwitz got around the problem by always wearing long sleeves. The Israeli novelist David Grossman tells the story of his own wedding, when a relative of the bride, anxious not to mar such a happy occasion by upsetting the guests, covered hers with a Band-Aid.

Later, in her Toronto shop, Catherine sometimes thought of those shivering naked women she had seen in Auschwitz, all their bodily imperfections on display. And as a saleswoman, seeing her customers in the changing room with all their flaws and faults, stripped down to their underwear, she wanted to clothe them, to cover them up, to conceal from hostile and unforgiving eyes their too-broad hips and sagging breasts. She understood implicitly, through this deep experience in her past which the customer knew nothing about, the therapeutic motive in shopping for clothes.

❦

One morning Catherine, ever dazzling in one of her Lacroix jackets, told me a story about an incident which had taken place the day before, at Holt Renfrew, where she had gone to try to find shoes on sale. But the story really began sixty years earlier, on a street in Rome, the Via Veneto, where she stood before the window of a shoe shop, and saw a pair of black suede high-heeled shoes. She was with a man from the Joint, the Jewish refugee agency, and watching the hunger on her face for beautiful shoes, he took her inside to buy them.

But she had been carrying rails in the snow at the satellite camp at Auschwitz. Her feet were still distorted and swollen. "Even though the Italian shoes are wide, nothing fitted me. I think my shoe size had changed. I was so hungry, I was standing with this man in a bar, and they had all these salamis, and he said, 'Have something to eat,' and I wanted to have everything. I just was eating, eating, and then he took me to the shoe shop, but the eating was more successful—I never did get the shoes."

That evening, after the attempt to buy shoes at the Holt Renfrew sale, she was having cocktails with a friend, a woman in her thirties, and it turned out she, too, had been trying on shoes at Holt that afternoon; in fact, Catherine had seen the discarded shoes of an earlier customer and asked to try them in her size. And it must have been this same woman because they had both been looking at exactly the same shoes: Roger Vivier, Prada, Chloé, Jimmy Choo.

The two women, several decades apart in age, bemoaned what had happened to shoe design. Neither of them could walk a step, so high were the heels.

Catherine had been delighted that, when she'd pointed to the pile of shoes on the floor and asked the sales girl to find them in her size, the girl had not tactfully said something about these being young women's shoes. "I was amazed. When I had my shop I would have said, I don't know that these shoes would fit you. But she went for half an hour looking for the size. And then I got up from the chair and I couldn't even walk towards the mirror in them, the heels were so high.

"I thought about Rome and I said to myself, Isn't it an irony of justice that even now I still have the desire for these fancy shoes, but still they don't fit me! It was a comedy. What is amazing is that the shoe designers today, they are putting this trauma on women. I don't know how this happened and this is not going to stay because there were hundreds of shoes reduced and they can't sell them because nobody can walk in them.

"There I was in Holt's, thinking about Rome, and my feet are fine, really, but I was thinking, Here I am, sixty years later, and now I can't wear these shoes. I can't even complain that the Germans did that to me.

"You know, happiness is so fleeting. The moments that you have the highs, at the peak of the mountain, it's so wonderful. I guess I am blessed because I know the difference. I have experienced the difference between the sorrow and the joy—there is such extremity in my life. Still, I am amazed that I was able to come from the ashes. And there is still my hope and my idealism. I feel confident that I'm going to live a long time. I feel I have a young soul."

Do not look upon all this that I am telling about the clothes as uncalled for or spun out, for they have a great deal to do with the story.

∞ MIGUEL DE CERVANTES

POSTSCRIPT

PEOPLE WILL ALWAYS tell you that they feel themselves to be old souls, but how many tell you that their soul is young? How old is Catherine? I know but won't tell. She's right, it doesn't matter. A teenager in Auschwitz, then sitting out the 1950s as an unhappy wife, beginning her career in the 1960s, discovering Armani, Ferre, and Versace in the 1970s—work it out yourself if you need to. But bear in mind that today I got an e-mail from a mutual friend who had dinner with her last night. Catherine is taking her fitness regime in hand, having signed up to a new program at Florida Jacks Boxing Club.

Catherine *is* fashion. She is fashion's agelessness, its ability always to occupy the present tense, and the opportunity it offers us all to reinvent ourselves. She understands, from dark experience, our need to be clothed, our desire for pleasure and for beauty in our lives. She embodies all of fashion's dynamic exhibitionism, its excess, its understanding of form and harmony and how you disturb it to create something new. This knowledge comes from deep inside her and from her journey through life, with all its terrors and its joys.

Since meeting her, I have learned to only buy what I love and what is life enhancing, regardless of its cost. Last week I had gone shopping with my friend who has the fabric friends to comfort her in her new foreign posting. Who refuses ever to buy high street. I wanted to show her a coat I was interested in at Jaeger, a blown-up hound's-tooth design with balloon sleeves. We met first for lunch at a department store, with her little girl who is now two. On the way down the escalators I showed her a Gerard Darel coat I had tried on. It was hundreds of dollars cheaper than the Jaeger—perhaps it would do instead. It was not a love affair, but I thought it was a perfect example of a no-nonsense coat that was, as they say, a classic.

That? she said. Lacking her decisive eye, I had fallen into error. She gave me a short master class on what was wrong with the coat. The two buttons were too close together. The length was all wrong. It was not flattering. Embarrassed, I put it back on the hanger.

We wheeled the stroller up Regent Street to Jaeger. There was an evaluation. There was the point made that I would not get enough wear out of it because it was *too* special, and this had been my fear—that if I were to spend that much on a coat, then I would have to wear it all winter long for years on end, and then everyone would say, "Here she is in that bloody coat again." It was one thing to have a signature style, but quite another to be drearily dressed in the same thing which you could not accessorize because the fabric and the sleeves were making the shouty statement *Look at me*. You would need three or four coats to have this coat.

We left. I tried on coats by MaxMara but they bored me. In Nicole Farhi everything was a disaster. The little girl, meanwhile, found a pair of high-heeled shoes, pushed her plump feet into them, and made a confident clattering progress across the floor, to the amazement and delight of the staff and customers but not us. For she had already revealed her penchant for Difficult Shoes when she was bought a pair of jeweled and embroidered Aladdin's mules at the souk in Istanbul, aged seventeen months, and studiously practiced walking up and down the wooden floors of her apartment. Clomp, clomp.

Her mother bought a Vivienne Westwood dress at the sale. I was still empty-handed, and I thought that once I'd got rid of my censorious shopping companion I would go back and get that Jaeger coat, but before that we stepped into Armani.

You see a coat, you ask for it in your size. Not that coat, this coat and no other. And when they bring it to you, everyone turns around and looks, because the right coat, the right dress, the right hat is like a sneeze or an orgasm—there's no mistaking what has just happened.

"Wow," says your critical friend. *"Wow!"*

But the coat was half a size too small. Armani gave me a list of all their London retailers and sent me on a wild-goose chase all over London trying to find it, but no one had even heard of this particular coat. I was wild with anger, I was enraged and bitter and disappointed.

Later that evening my friend sent me a text. Her mother (who would shove copies of *Vogue* in her daughter's crib to keep her quiet, and the little girl would hold them, upside down, pretending to read) had been told all about this thwarted shopping trip. MY MOTHER SAYS THIS IS NOT THE END OF THE STORY.

I woke up the next morning thinking of the coat. That's how you know; your unconscious is perfectly rational when it comes to these things. I rang Armani and told them I would like to come and try it on again because you must never forget the possibility that the coat has grown an inch in the night, hanging alone in the darkness of the shut-up shop's stockroom. I have seen this happen before, though not normally to such a tight time scale.

That afternoon I walked up the stairs in my Dolce & Gabbana four-inch black patent heels to the dimly lit floor of women's wear, which seemed like a cathedral in which icons burned under the radiant dazzle of spotlights. There was music in the background; I heard priests singing and smelled the incense. I was close to divinity.

I put on the coat. It had not got any bigger in the night; no miracle had taken place, the miracle of the growing coat.

A willowy young man appeared with pins in his lapels and sleeves, fleeing across the floor like a gazelle, and stopped abruptly. *"Signora,"* he cried, "that coat is perfect for you!"

I felt tears of rage welling up inside me. "It's too small," I said.

"No, no," he replied. "We can do something. There is *always* something we can do." And he started to pin.

I looked at the price tag and winced. But I remembered Catherine and I remembered all the once-beloved red shoes. Take pleasure, I thought, take it while you can.

ACKNOWLEDGMENTS

Above all, I would like to thank Catherine Hill for agreeing to share with me her extraordinary story, and for the many insights I have taken from our intense mornings together about fashion. The full story of Catherine's remarkable life will be told one day in her own book, which she is writing. The utmost gratitude, too, to Robert Jan van Pelt and Miriam Greenbaum, for first suggesting that the two of us should meet, and for opening their own home to a stranger. Their warm and generous hospitality made the trip to Toronto possible. Anthony Julius made the introduction in the first place, when I asked him about the red shoes. I'm grateful to Avsh Alom Gur for explaining the whole business of sexy.

I am indebted to the many readers of my blog, "The Thoughtful Dresser," which I established as a means of thinking aloud about clothes in November 2007. Across the world, in the Nevada desert, in Algeria, Saudi Arabia, Hong Kong, Australia, Oslo, and many other places, there are intelligent women who are interested in clothes. My heartfelt thanks to those who contributed to my question about fashion after 9/11, and whose comments I have reproduced here.

A great number of the quotations and aphorisms are taken from a little book I bought some years ago and which has been my constant companion ever since: Tobi Tobias's *Obsessed by Dress* (Beacon Press, 2000).

Thanks to my indefatigable agent, Derek Johns; my editor, Lennie Goodings (both of whom always get it); and the whole team at Little Brown, especially Susan de Soissons.

About the Author

Linda Grant was born in Liverpool and now lives in London. Her first novel, *The Cast Iron Shore*, won the David Higham First Novel Prize and was shortlisted for the *Guardian* Fiction Prize. Her second novel, *When I Lived in Modern Times*, won the Orange Prize for Fiction. *Still Here* was nominated for the Man Booker Prize. Linda Grant is also the author of *Sexing the Millennium: A Political History of the Sexual Revolution*; *Remind Me Who I Am, Again*, a family memoir; and *The People on the Street: A Writer's View of Israel*, which won the Lettre Ulysses Award for Literary Reportage. Her novel *The Clothes on Their Backs* was shortlisted for the Man Booker Prize 2008.